Growing Your Own
Living Foods

Brian Hetrich

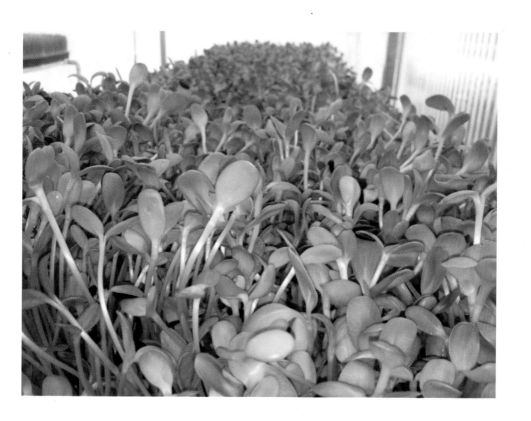

"Sprouting The Easy Way"

Publisher
New Life Books

Photography
New Life Books

Cover Art, Design, Layout & Editing
New Life Books

Medical Disclaimer:
The food and health information in this book is based upon the training, experience, and research of the authors and is intended to inform and educate. It is not intended to diagnose, treat, or cure any disease. Check with a qualified health professional prior to beginning this or any health program. The author and publisher specifically disclaim any liability, loss, risk, personal or otherwise which is incurred as a consequence, directly or indirectly, of the use and application of the contents of this book.

ISBN: 9780692600559

Acknowledgement

I would like to thank the person that introduced me to raw foods, Dr. Jim Sharps. In 2005, I attended a lecture by Dr. Sharps on "Healthy Living" which opened my mind. His example, wise counsel, and motivation inspired me and cast me off on an absolutely amazing health journey that has completely turned my life around for the better.

- Brian Hetrich

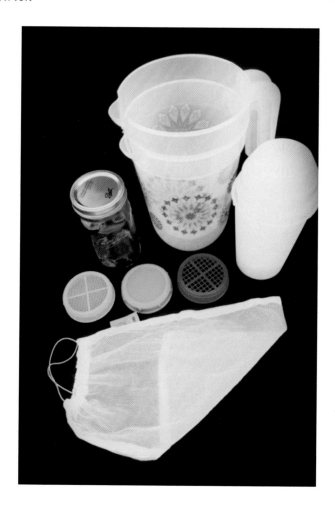

Table of Contents

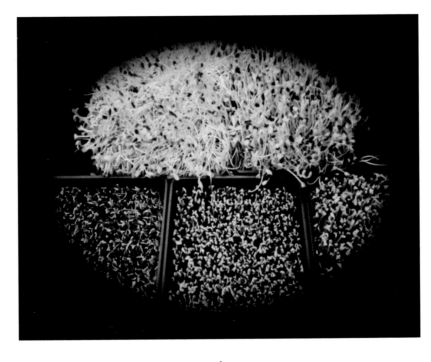

"About the Author"

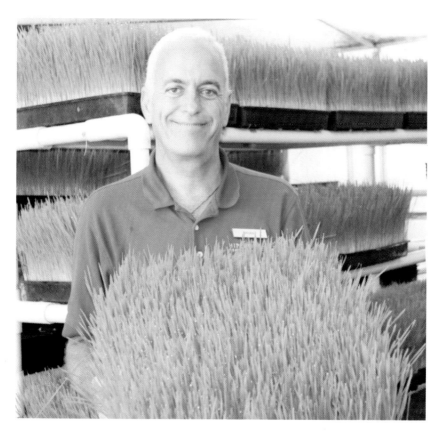

<u>Brian Hetrich</u>

I lived most of my life eating the Standard American Diet (SAD.) As a result of this eating habit I developed many of the ailments of the typical American person. I became seriously overweight, I was "tired all the time", and developed a whole host of chronic ailments including headaches, backaches, high blood pressure, high cholesterol, I was sick all the time), low energy, allergies, acne, poor vision, brain fog, poor sleep to name a few. I reluctantly accepted this as normal because the same thing seemed to be happening to almost everybody else. Finally, I became just plain sick and tired of being sick and tired. I tried every kind of diet and exercise I could think of, and nothing worked. I began searching for a change.

Growing Your Own Living Foods

In January 2005 I attended a lecture on health given by a very fit-looking naturopath, Dr. Jim Sharps. Something he said caught my attention - he mentioned raw foods and claimed that going on a "raw food diet" was the most amazing thing he had ever done in his life. I found his presentation very compelling and inspirational. I decided to make some small changes to my meals and began to move towards a more plant-based diet. I went vegetarian for a year then, vegan for a year and then "high raw" for another year. Each step of the way I noticed more and more improvements to my health. I was very intrigued by these positive changes and decided to go 100% raw just to see what would happen.

I simply cannot overemphasize the power of raw foods! To say that going from SAD to 100% raw is like "night and day" is an understatement. It is more like being launched to another reality or dimension! Not only did I quickly lose 100 pounds of excess weight but, all of my health challenges went away and my mental clarity, focus, awareness, sensitivity and sense of connectedness soared to levels I never knew existed! Without me realizing it this new found sense of awareness and energy began to steer my life in another direction.

Upon graduating from the International Institute of Original Medicine (IIOM) as a Doctor of Naturopathy in Original Medicine, I started my own private practice in Maryland, hosting Raw Food Retreats, began to teach gourmet raw food "cooking" classes, host raw potlucks, raw chocolate parties, movie nights and health education lectures. IIOM is accredited by the American Naturopathic Medical Accreditation Board (ANMAB), and the American Association of Drugless Practitioners (AADP.) I also co-authored the book, "Natural Vibrant Health – Raw Foods" which is a collection of my favorite raw food recipes. My book is available online and in the Hippocrates store.

I am now responsible for growing all the wheatgrass, sprouts, herbs, fruits, and vegetables at The Hippocrates Health Institute in West Palm Beach, Florida. I am a key part of the Hippocrates educational experience for guests at the institute. My classes teach Life Transformation Program and Health Educator Program participants essential information including: growing sprouts and wheatgrass, juicing, organic gardening, and water purification.

Growing Your Own Living Foods

I earned my Bachelor of Science degree in Business Administration from Towson University with a specific focus on leadership and management. I have many years of experience in the business world as sales manager for national accounts. I have Six Sigma Greenbelt Certification and been extensively trained in professional selling and high impact presentation skills for large corporate audiences. I have a Universal EPA Certification from the Refrigeration Environmental Protection Association. I also have an ASE Refrigerant Recovery & Recycling Certification from the Society of Automotive Engineers. I have been trained in High Impact Presentations and Leadership from Dale Carnegie Seminars. I have been inducted into one of my previous employer's prestigious President's Club for consistent exceptional performance.

I have been 100% raw vegan since 2007. In my free time I enjoy gardening, hiking, camping, biking, art, music, yoga, chi gong, exercise, ballroom dancing, walking on the beach, and cars.

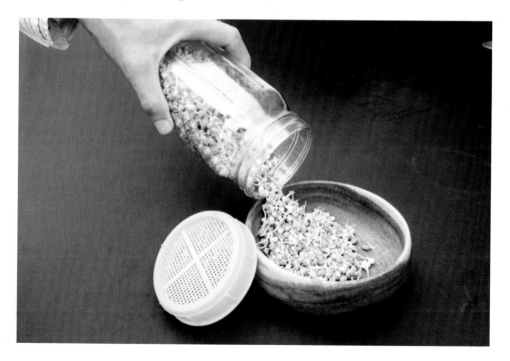

Growing Your Own Living Foods

Growing Your Own Living Foods

<u>Chapter 1 –Why Sprouts?</u>

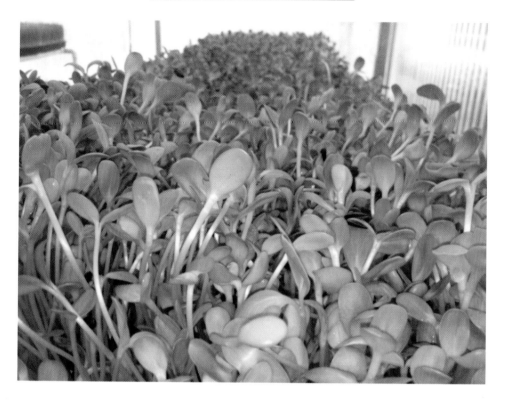

Sprouting is easy - and anybody can do it!
Here are just some of the many reasons to grow your own living foods:

- **Nutrition:** Sprouts are the most nutritious whole food on the planet. This is high frequency, high vibration living food that conveys its life-force energy to you!
- **Economics:** Sprout seeds multiply to 3-20 times their weight. You can feed yourself and your family the most nutritious organic food on the planet for under a dollar a pound.. You can grow five pounds of food in the form of sprouts in one square foot of kitchen countertop space.
- **Organic:** There is no need to use any artificial chemicals, pesticides, herbicides, or fungicides.

- **Freshness:** Sprouts are the ultimate in freshness because you can pick and eat them the same day. There is virtually no loss of nutrients.
- **Variety:** Any edible plant can be eaten as a sprout. And, there are thousands of them! These are baby plants in their prime at the peak of their nutrition and at the peak of their flavor. Every plant mines different minerals as it grows. By having a variety of sprouts in your diet you can get a balanced nutritional profile.
- **Emergency Preparedness:** Sprout seeds can last a really long time if tightly sealed and stored in a cool, dry environment.

Medicinally and nutritionally, sprouts have a long history as a "health" food. Sprouts are **10 to 30 times** more nutritious than the best vegetables because they are baby plants in their prime. At this stage of their growth they have the greatest concentration of nutrients than at any other point in their life. Sprouts are highly digestible and release their nutrients easily due to their delicate cell walls and abundance of enzymes.

When you apply water to seeds they come to life. By the natural process of transmutation, the vitamin, mineral, enzyme, phytonutrient, and amino acid (protein) content of germinated (sprouted) foods skyrocket! This phenomenon is most pronounced during the first twelve days of growth. This makes sprouts a true "superfood." They are also biogenic and alive. Biogenic foods are foods that create new life when planted. Sprouts are alive and this life-force energy is capable of transferring their life energy to your body.

Germination unleashes dormant vitamins, minerals, and enzymes that make them on average ten to thirty times more nutritious than even the best raw, organically-grown vegetables. The enzyme content in sprouts is up to 100 times higher than raw vegetables. Certain B-vitamins increase 1200 percent during the germination process. Because of this super concentration of natural enzymes, sprouts are more easily digestible and the nutrients are more bio-available. Full of antioxidants and a full profile of enzymes, vitamins and minerals, sprouts make the perfect living food. Because sprouts also contain an abundance of highly-active antioxidants that prevent DNA destruction that protect us from the ongoing effects of aging and cellular breakdown, recent research shows they can also have an important curative ability as well. Sprouts like alfalfa, radish, broccoli, clover and mung bean contain concentrated amounts of phytochemicals that can protect against disease. Johns Hopkins University found that broccoli sprouts contain a substance called sulforaphane, a compound that helps mobilize the body's natural cancer-fighting resources and reduces risk of developing cancer. In fact their research determined that broccoli sprouts are the most powerful anti-cancer substance ever discovered – either natural or man-made.[1]

Sprouts also contain a high source of fiber, are easily digestible and contain a high concentration of enzymes facilitating the digestive process. Many sprouts also contain plant estrogens, which have been shown to help increase bone formation and density, prevent bone breakdown or osteoporosis, and can be helpful in controlling hot flashes, menopause, PMS symptoms and fibrocystic breast tumors. Likewise, studies on canavanine -- an amino acid found in alfalfa -- have been shown to fight certain types of cancers, including pancreatic, colon and leukemia cancers.[2] Alfalfa sprouts are also a good source of saponins, which lower the bad cholesterol and fat but not the good HDL fats, and also stimulate the immune system by increasing the activity of natural killer cells such as T- lymphocytes and interferon. Interestingly, the saponin content of alfalfa sprouts is more than 400 percent over that of an un-sprouted seed.

[1]Angier, Natalie (1997-09-16). "Researchers Find a Concentrated Anticancer Substance in Broccoli Sprouts" – The New York Times.

[2]Green, M.H., Brooks, T.L., Mendelsohn, J., and Howell, S.B., (1980). Antitumor activity of L-canavanine against L1210 murine leukemia. *Cancer Res.* 40: 535-537.

Growing Your Own Living Foods

Chapter 2 - Sprout Types

There are over 250,000 known edible plant species on this planet. All of them can be eaten as a baby geminated seed or, what we call a "sprout." All edibles are highly nutritious in the sprouted form. Listed here are twenty different types of sprouts chosen primarily upon their popularity, availability of the seeds, and their great medicinal value.

Adzuki

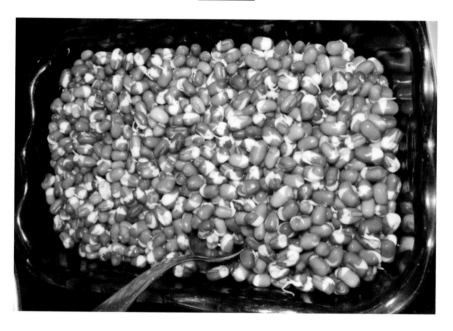

Origin:
- Far East

Health Benefits:
- Energy
- Protein
- Lowers LDL cholesterol
- Regulates insulin
- Fights breast and colon cancer

<u>Alfalfa</u>

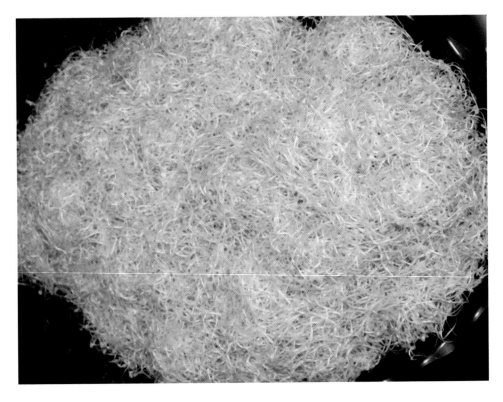

Origin:
- South-Central Asia

Health Benefits:
- Blood builder
- Relaxes the nervous system
- Settles the stomach and treats throat and stomach cancer
- An excellent expectorant - treats whooping cough
- Promotes fertility

Growing Your Own Living Foods

<u>Chinese Bean Sprouts</u>

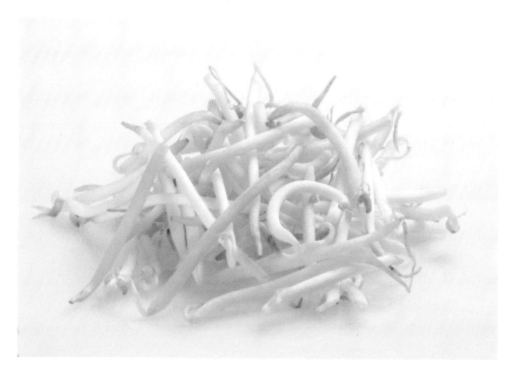

Origin:
- Far East

Health Benefits:
- Energy
- Protein
- Helps prevent prostate problems and glandular dysfunction
- Helps prevent breast cancer
- Helps with premature balding and graying

Beet Sprouts

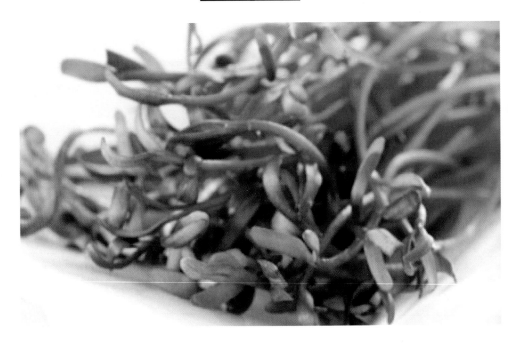

Origin:
- Mediterranean region

Health Benefits:
- Blood builder
- Digestion
- Aphrodisiac and a natural Viagra
- Human sex hormones

Growing Your Own Living Foods

<u>Broccoli</u>

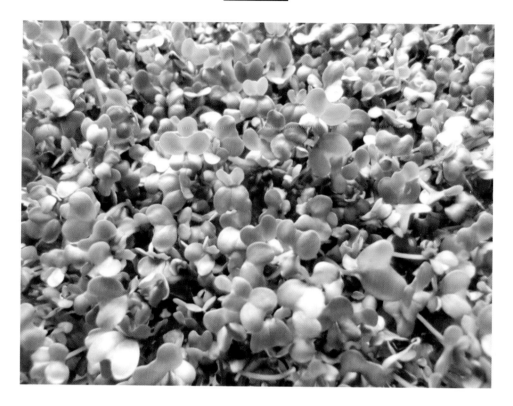

Origin:
- Northern and western Mediterranean region

Health Benefits:
- Helps fight colon, prostate, rectum, esophagus, lung, bladder, and stomach cancer
- Effective for inflammations and hot swellings
- Effective for hangovers

Growing Your Own Living Foods

Buckwheat

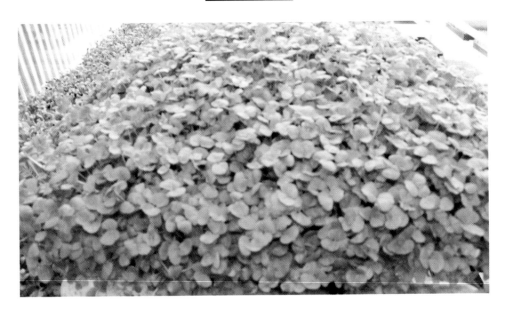

Origin:
- Southeast Asia

Health Benefits:
- Protein
- Lowers high blood pressure
- Blood sugar balancer
- Good for varicose veins
- Helps prevent osteoporosis
- Helps prevent anxiety, depression, brain fog, mental fatigue and generally make the brain sharper and clearer.

Cabbage

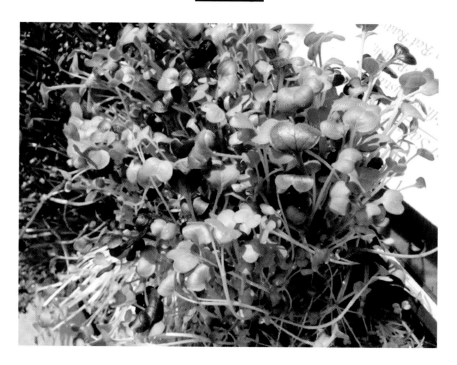

Origin:
- Britain and continental Europe

Health Benefits:
- Helps fight colon, prostate, rectum, esophagus, lung, bladder, and stomach cancer
- Effective for inflammations and hot swellings
- Effective for hangovers

<u>Chia Sprouts</u>

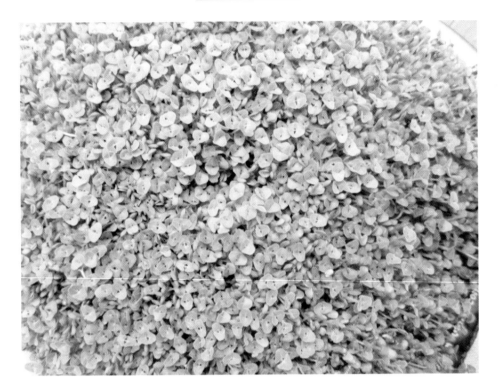

Origin:
- Central and South America

Health Benefits:
- Omega-3 EFA's
- Energy
- Protein
- Blood sugar balancer
- Reduces inflammation
- Enhances cognitive performance
- Reduces high cholesterol
- Calcium, Manganese, Magnesium, Phosphorus, Zinc, Vitamin B3 (Niacin), Potassium, Vitamin B1 (Thiamine) and Vitamin B2.

Clover

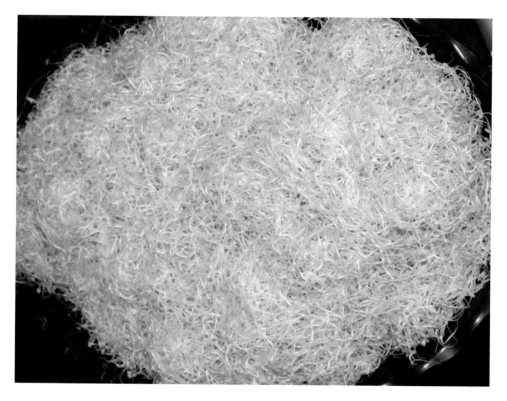

Origin:
- Northern Hemisphere

Health Benefits:
- Blood builder
- Heart and cardiovascular health
- Strong bones
- Anti-cancer, Anti-aging

Fenugreek

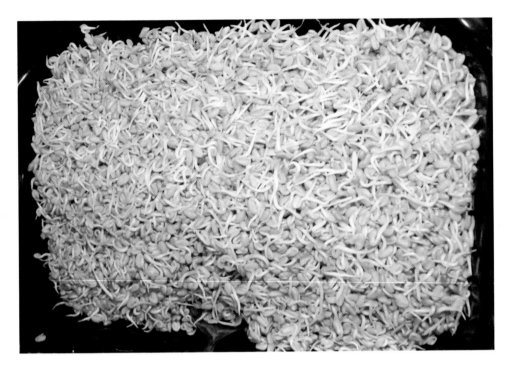

Origin:
- Mediterranean region

Health Benefits:
- Treats blood poisoning, failing eyesight, fevers, palpitations, liver and kidney troubles
- Treats anemia
- Blood sugar balancer
- Increases mother's milk production

<u>Flax</u>

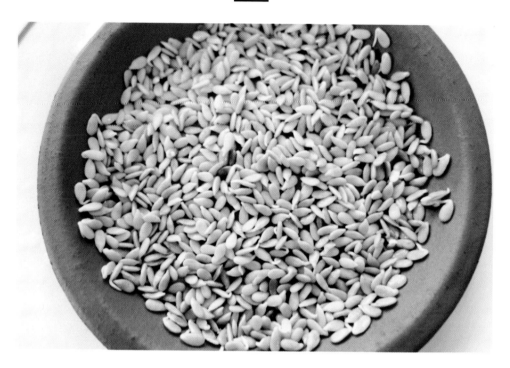

Origin:
- Mesopotamia

Health Benefits:
- Omega-3 EFA's
- Energy
- Protein
- Blood sugar balancer
- Calcium, Manganese, Magnesium, Phosphorus, Zinc, Vitamin B3 (Niacin), Potassium, Vitamin B1 (Thiamine) and Vitamin B2.

Garbanzo

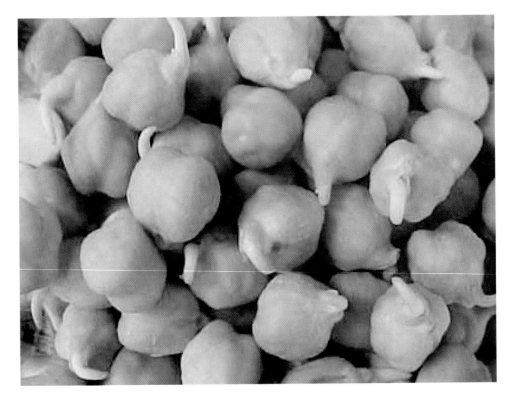

Origin:
- Middle East

Health Benefits:
- Protein
- Energy
- Blood sugar balancer
- Lowers blood cholesterol

Growing Your Own Living Foods

<u>Garlic Sprouts</u>

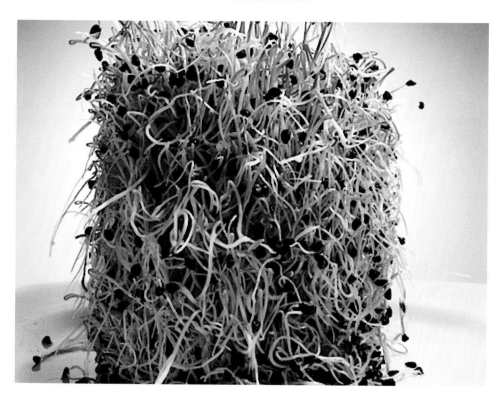

Origin:
- Central Asia

Health Benefits:
- Heart health
- Helps fight against cancer
- Helps prevent wrinkles and premature aging
- Boosts the immune system

<u>Green Lentils</u>

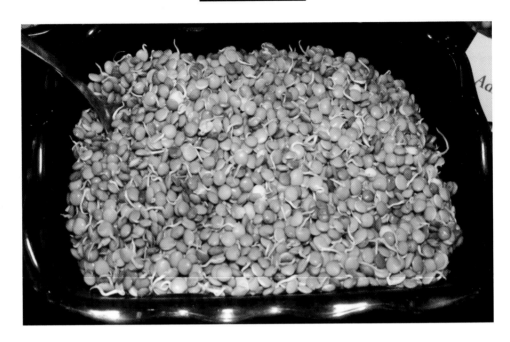

Origin:
- Mediterranean region

Health Benefits:
- Energy
- Protein
- Lowers LDL cholesterol
- Regulates insulin
- Fights breast and colon cancer

Growing Your Own Living Foods

<u>Mung Beans</u>

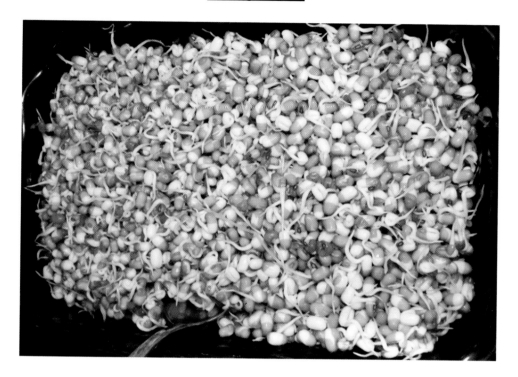

Origin:
- South-Central Asia

Health Benefits:
- Energy
- Helps prevent prostate problems.
- Helps prevent glandular dysfunction and breast cancer
- Treats premature balding

Onion Sprouts

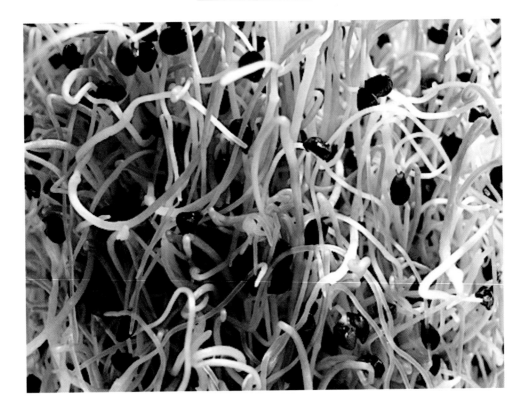

Origin:
- Central Asia

Health Benefits:
- Heart health
- Helps fight against cancer
- Helps prevent wrinkles and premature aging
- Boosts the immune system

Growing Your Own Living Foods

<u>Pea Shoots</u>

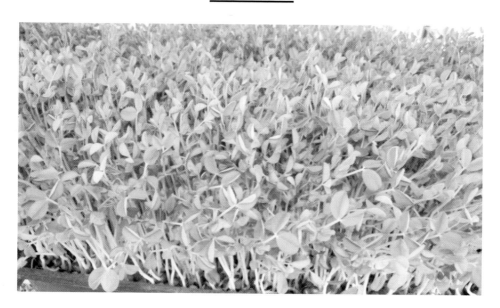

Origin:
- Mediterranean region

Health Benefits:
- Protein
- Muscle
- Strengthens teeth
- Boosts the immune system

<u>Radish</u>

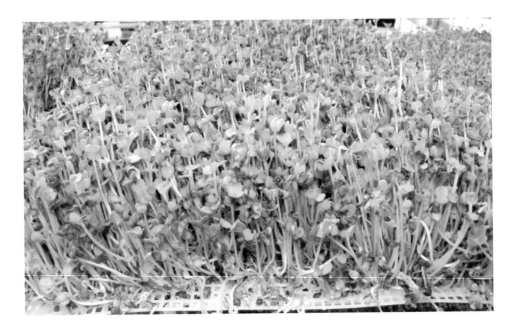

Origin:
- Western Asia

Health Benefits:
- Cleans the blood
- An excellent expectorant - treats whooping cough
- Facilitates digestion

Growing Your Own Living Foods

Red Lentils

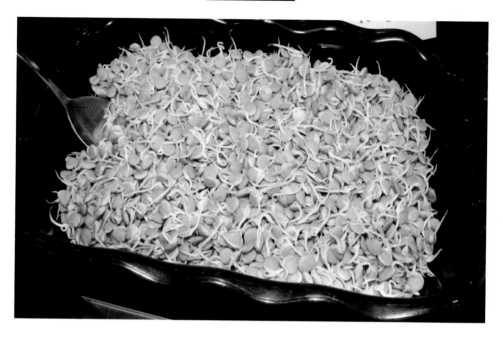

Origin:
- Mediterranean region

Health Benefits:
- Energy
- Protein
- Lowers LDL cholesterol
- Regulates insulin
- Fights breast and colon cancer

Growing Your Own Living Foods

<u>Sunflower</u>

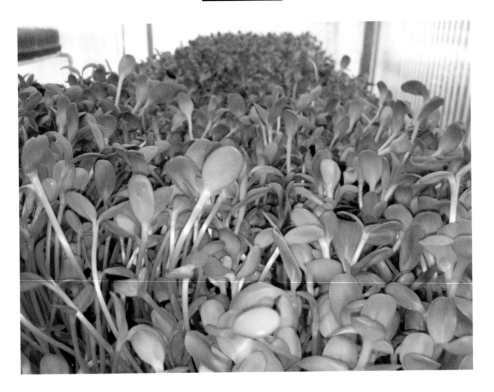

Origin:
- North America

Health Benefits:
- Excellent source of balanced amino acids for building protein
- Activates every cell in the immune system
- Builds skeletal, muscular and neurological systems
- A source of vitamin D.

Growing Your Own Living Foods

<u>Wheatgrass</u>

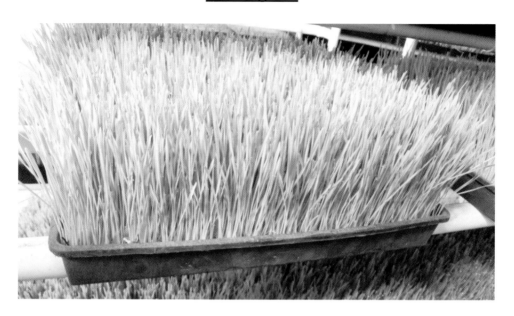

Origin:
- Mesopotamia

Health Benefits:
- Blood builder
- Anti-cancer
- Detoxifier
- Boosts the immune system

Growing Your Own Living Foods

Growing Your Own Living Foods

Chapter 3 – Getting Started

Sprouting is easy! Anybody can do it. Here is what you will need to get started growing sprouts:
1. Seeds
2. A sprouting vessel
3. Trays
4. Potting mix
5. A sprouting rack
6. A drain pan

You can do this without building a greenhouse. Believe it or not, the best place for you to grow all your sprouts is right in your own kitchen – for several different reasons.

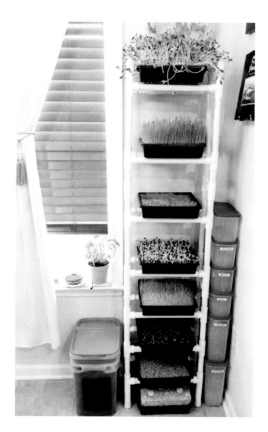

Growing Your Own Living Foods

Temperature

The temperature in your kitchen is perfect! Most people find between 65 and 75 degrees F (17-22 degrees C) to be a comfortable setting in their homes. This just so happens to be the ideal temperature to grow your sprouts. This means you can grow sprouts all year long regardless of where in the world you live because you always grow indoors.

Humidity

The humidity in your kitchen is perfect! The excess moisture in the air will condense on the evaporator coil while the air conditioner is running during the warmer months. This will automatically keep the humidity below 50% which is what sprouts prefer.

Lighting

The light level in your kitchen is perfect! Just leave the lights turned on twelve hours a day and turn them off at night. You want plenty of indirect sunlight and plenty of artificial light to supplement for cloudy days (full spectrum is better than conventional). However, you do not ever want any direct sunlight. If you have direct sunlight hitting any of your sprouts they will get too hot and they will cook. You need at least 1000 foot-candles. This is the same as 1000 lumens one foot away from the sprouts. If you have direct sunlight coming in the window hitting your sprouts just put a sheer curtain up or tint the glass in the window. That will diffuse the intensity of the sunlight just enough so it will not cook your sprouts.

Ventilation

A little bit of gentle air flow is desirable. A ceiling fan on "low" somewhere nearby in the room is ideal. You could also use a pedestal fan or a tabletop fan. If you see the blades of grass moving as a result of the action of the fan then it is too high or it is too close. Just move the fan further away or use a lower fan speed setting.

Growing Your Own Living Foods

Water Source

The kitchen is also the best place to grow all your sprouts because you have a water source right in the same room at the kitchen sink. Remember, you will be watering twice a day - so you want to make this easy and convenient. You want to use fresh, filtered water for each soak and rinse. The ZeroWater pitcher filter is very effective at filtering water and is reasonably priced. You can find the ZeroWater pitcher at Bed, Bath and Beyond, Target, and Kmart.

Space Requirements

Sprouting really does not require a lot of space. You can grow five pounds of food in the form of sprouts in one square foot of kitchen countertop space. This takes care of all the beans, legumes, and leafy sprouts. Using a tiered rack such as the seven-tiered Hydrosol rack, you can grow all the wheatgrass, sunflower, buckwheat and pea shoot sprouts you need for two people in two square feet of floor space. You can have a nice butcher block cutting board cut to size to fit over your stovetop and use that area for growing sprouts.

Focal Point

The kitchen is also the best place to grow because that is where we tend to spend most of our time in our houses outside of the bedroom. The kitchen is where we tend to congregate because that is where the food is☺! You want to make your sprout growing operation the new focal point of your life because this could change your life☺!

The sprouts you are growing will get a lot of attention from the guests you are entertaining and will be a great topic of conversation. People generally know that sprouts are good for you and they will be fascinated with your new project. Your friends and family will be curious as to why you have suddenly become so healthy and why you are so radiant. They will be interested in learning how to do it for themselves. Sprouts are beautiful! Sprouts are full of life! Sprouts clean the air! You will be proud of your progress and you want your sprouts to be front and center for all to see!

Growing Your Own Living Foods

When you take all of these things into consideration, there is no question that the best place to grow your sprouts is right in your own kitchen.

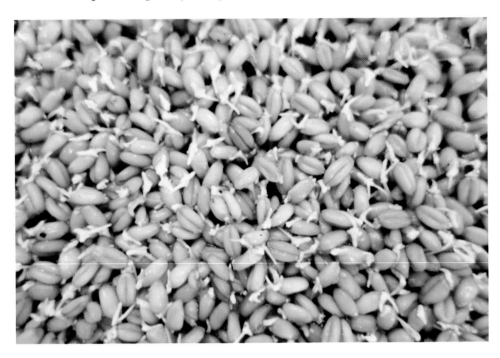

Chapter 4 - Seeds

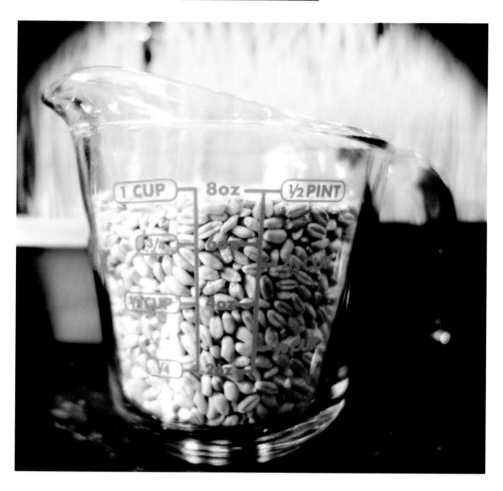

The first thing you will need in order to get started sprouting are obviously the seeds. Not all seeds are created equal. <u>You will want to be sure your seeds are 100% organic and they are commercially distributed with the intention of sprouting.</u> They must be whole, raw, fresh, and not heat processed, pasteurized, or irradiated.

If you go to your local grocery store you will find beans and legumes in the soup isle. However, these seeds are sold with the intention of making soups and stews. Chances are they may have been:

Growing Your Own Living Foods

1. Pasteurized
2. Heat processed
3. Irradiated
4. Crushed (such as rolled oats)
5. Split (such as split peas)
6. Cut (such as steel cut oats)

All of the above processes kill the life force energy in the seeds and will prevent them from sprouting. If you intend to make soup or stew, this is irrelevant since the seeds will be cooked. However, you're not reading this book to learn how to make soup - you want to start sprouting!

Seed Sources:
1. Online at Jaffe Brothers http://organicfruitsandnuts.com, a sprout house such as "Got Sprouts" http://www.gotsprouts.com or "Universal Living Sprouts" http://www.ulsprouts.com or Handy Pantry https://www.handypantry.com/
2. A "hard core" health food store in your home town. An example in West Palm Beach, Florida is "Nutrition Smart."
3. The Hippocrates Health Institute store https://www.hippocratesstore.org. All seeds sold here are 100% organic and are carefully selected for the best performance.

Seeds have a shelf life. They will last for a few hours or a few years depending upon the type of seed and the amount of exposure to heat, humidity, and bugs. When you purchase your seeds, keep them cool and dry. Don't leave them sitting in the car while you do other shopping or run more errands. The temperature in your car will quickly get above 160 degrees F while parked in the hot sun. This might kill some of your seeds. Treat your seeds like supplements. Take them home right away or use a cooler with ice.

Seeds are often sold in plastic bags, which is fine if you plan on using them in a few months. If you plan on keeping them longer than that you should transfer them out of plastic bags and into dry glass containers with a tight sealing lid with a gasket (such a Mason jar). If you leave your seeds

Growing Your Own Living Foods

in plastic bags, bugs will eventually eat right through the plastic to get to them. Keep your seeds in the pantry at room temperature. Better yet, keep them in the refrigerator if you have space. However, you do not want to store them in the freezer - doing so will kill them.

Different seeds have different shelf lives. For example, if kept dry and in tightly sealed glass containers your seeds will last approximately:

Seed Type	40 degrees F. Refrigerator	80 degrees F. Room temperature	100 degrees F. Outside (summer)
Alfalfa	8 years	12 months	2.25 months
Clover	8 years	12 months	2.25 months
Radish	7 years	10.5 months	2 months
Broccoli	6 years	9 months	1.75 months
Adzuki	5 years	7.5 months	1.5 months
Peas	5 years	7.5 months	1.5 months
Garbanzo	5 years	7.5 months	1.5 months
Lentils	4 years	6 months	1 month
Mung	4 years	6 months	1 month
Wheat	4 years	6 months	1 month
Sunflower	2 years	3 months	18 days

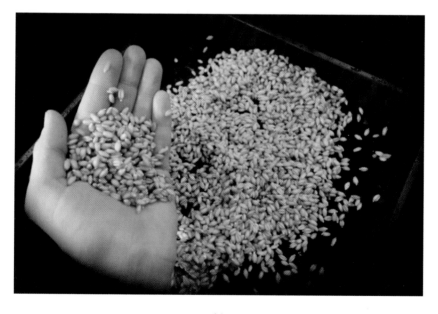

Growing Your Own Living Foods

Chapter 5 - Sprouting Vessels

The next thing you will need is a sprouting vessel. This will be used for soaking and rinsing the seeds. There are several types of sprouting vessels that can be used interchangeably. Each one has its own pros and cons. Here are a few examples:

Mason Jars with Sprouting Lids

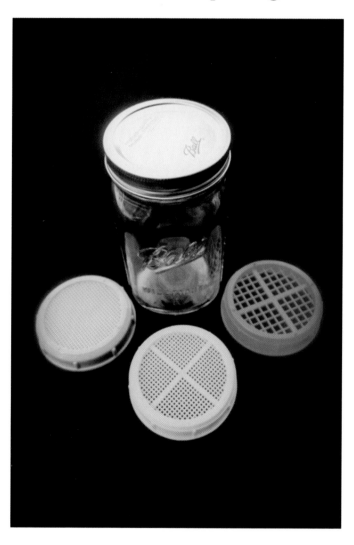

Growing Your Own Living Foods

A one quart wide mouth Mason jar is my favorite choice as a sprouting vessel and this is the one that most experienced sprouters eventually return to. The jar is made of glass which is an excellent alternative to plastic if you would like to reduce your toxic exposure. Mason jars are also readily available at any place that sells canning supplies. People use them for canning or for making pickles, sauerkraut, jams, jellies, and preserves. Typically, Kmart, Target, Whole Foods, and Walmart will carry these year-round or in some cases seasonally in the fall. Mason jars are also very versatile. In addition to being used as a sprouting vessel they can also be used for dry seed storage, and for drinking juices or smoothies. Mason jars are heavy glass and are relatively inexpensive, about $1.00 apiece.

Sprout lids can be purchased at any good hardcore health food store or the Hippocrates Health Institute store or online. The sprout lids are about $3.00 apiece. So, for $4.00 you are in business. My favorite type are called Toppers made by Sprout-Ease. They come in three colors: yellow, green, and red. The yellow lid has small holes in it for small seeds like alfalfa, clover and broccoli. The green lid has medium holes in it for medium sized seeds like mung beans, lentils, and wheatgrass. The red lids are for large seeds like sunflower and garbanzo. You can also use the red lids and Mason jars for soaking your pecans, almonds, and walnuts. You want to make sure that all your nuts and seeds are raw and that you soak them in water for eight hours before you eat them and use them in recipes. This makes them easier to digest and more nutritious.

Toppers also have tiny little plastic nubs on top of the lids which act as stand-offs. So, even when you have your jars directly upside down on a flat surface such as the base of your sink or a drain pan, these stand-offs create a small gap so air can get underneath the jar and inside so the sprouts can breathe.

Growing Your Own Living Foods

Mason Jars with Cheese Cloth

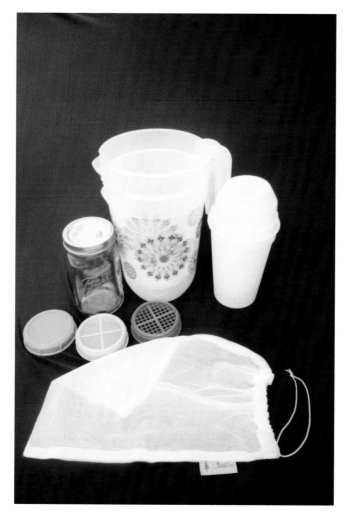

As an alternative to sprout lids you could use a one-quart wide mouth Mason jar and drape a 6" X 6" piece of cheesecloth or fabric screen material over the mouth of the jar and then thread the outer rim of the jar lid over the top of the fabric. The benefit of cheese cloth is that it is easier to find compared to sprout lids and they cost less. So, for little more than the cost of a Mason jar you are in business! However, the cheese cloth will not last as long as the sprout lids and they are a little harder to keep clean.

Growing Your Own Living Foods

Sprout bags

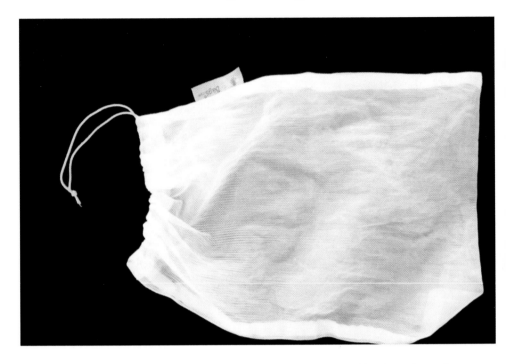

Sprout bags fold up flat taking up almost no space at all. Plus, there is no glass to break. This makes them an excellent choice for travelling, camping or hiking.

Growing Your Own Living Foods

Pitcher Method

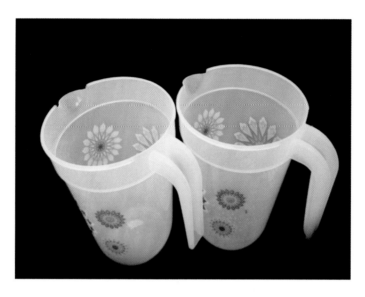

The pitcher method offers the option of growing lager batches of sprouts since the pitchers are available in increased capacities such as two or four quarts. Plus, you can use the pitcher method to grow the popular thick-rooted Chinese bean sprouts. The type of pitcher to use is a standard restaurant "water service" pitcher. Some people call these Cool Aid pitchers or beer pitchers. The secret is to find pitchers that are "stackable" where the handle is open on one end so they can sleeve inside one another. You may find these at Target, Wal-Mart, K-Mart, a restaurant supply store and sometimes at the dollar store. You will need at least two of these pitchers in the two quart size or larger.

In order to use the pitcher method you will need to modify one of them by drilling holes in the bottom. Just place one of the pitchers upside down on a table and drill about 30 holes in the bottom with a drill and the appropriately sized drill bit for the type of sprout you intend to grow.

Seed Size	Type	Drill Bit Size
Small	alfalfa, clover, broccoli, etc.	1/16"
Medium	mung, lentil, adzuki, wheat	5/32"
Large	Sunflower, garbanzo, etc.	¼"

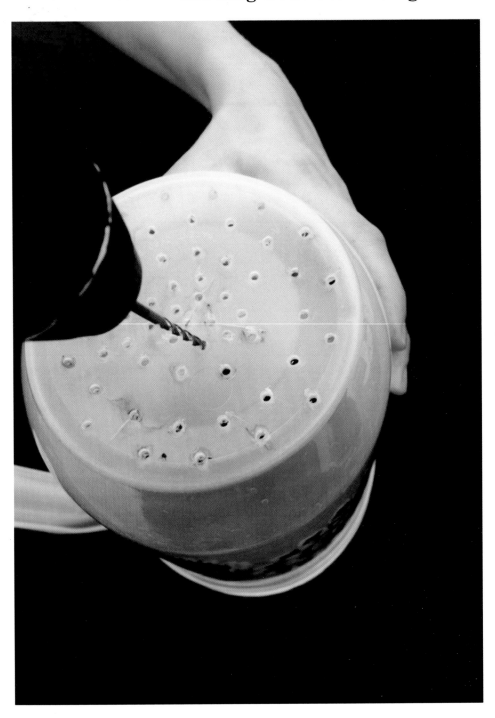

Growing Your Own Living Foods

EasySprouter

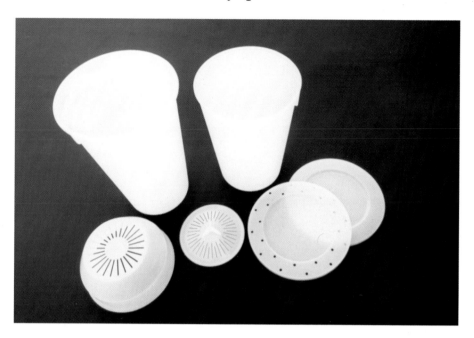

The EasySprout sprouter has a unique feature that cuts your sprouting time in half. This is accomplished by employing a clever design that produces a "chimney effect" inside your sprouter. This works like the flue in a home fireplace, introducing more air into the growing equation. As the sprouts grow they create a miniscule amount of heat. As the heat rises inside the sprouter, it flows out of the vent holes in the top of the domed lid. This creates a draft which draws more air in the vent holes in the bottom of the inner cup. This is all made possible by the air gap that is created between the inner and the outer cup by lifting and turning the inner cup so that it sits up on the top ledge on the outer cup.

There are six separate parts to the EasySprout sprouter:
- A solid lid for storage.
- A lid with holes in it for travelling.
- A measuring cup with holes in the bottom. When inverted it doubles as a domed lid which creates the chimney effect.

- An inner cup which has holes in the bottom and ribs around the perimeter of the top.
- An outer cup which has keyways around the perimeter of the top.
- A small seed insert which snaps in the bottom of the inner cup to prevent small seeds from draining out of the cup along with the soak and rinse water.

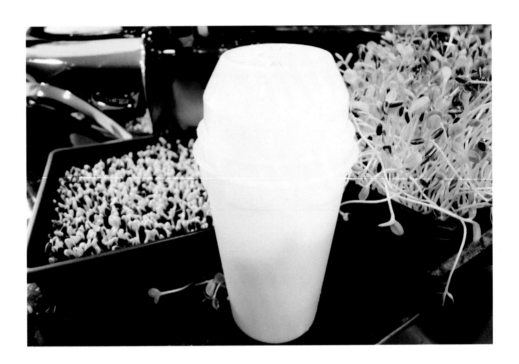

Chapter 6 – Soaking and Rinsing

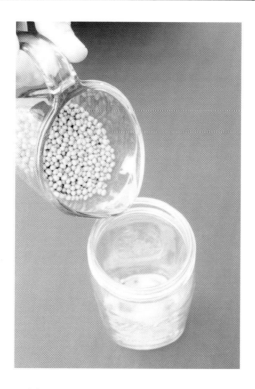

All sprouting starts with soaking. This dramatically increases the germination rate of the dry seeds. Soaking simulates the rain fall which wakes the seed up and tells it that it is time to grow. For soaking you can use any one of the sprouting vessels discussed in the previous chapter. They all work equally well for this function.

Sprout Vessel Type	Soaking
Sprout jar	Add seeds and water inside the jar and screw on the sprout lid.
Sprout bag	Add seeds to the bag and submerse in a bowl of water.
Pitcher method	Add seeds inside the pitcher with holes and sleeve inside a regular unmodified pitcher. Add water.
EasySprouter	Add seeds to the inner cup and sleeve inside the outer cup. Add water.

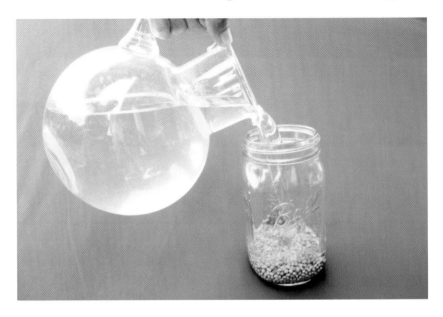

For soaking use at least three parts water to one part seed. Use fresh, filtered water. You can't have too much water but, you can have too little. If you start soaking with not enough water the seeds may rise above the soak water as they begin to germinate and swell in size.

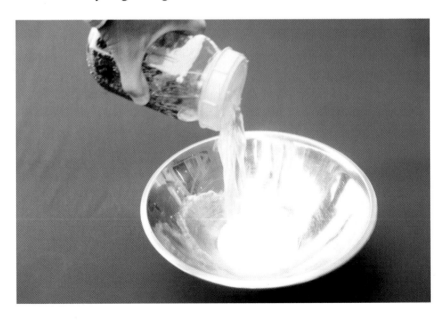

Growing Your Own Living Foods

Here are the recommended seed quantities, lid colors, soak time, and rinse times for two dozen different types of sprouts.

Seed Type	Dry Measure	Lid Color	Soak Time
Adzuki beans	½ cup	green	12 hours
Alfalfa	2 tsp.	yellow	4 hours
Almonds	as needed	red	8 hours
Amaranth	½ cup	yellow	3 hours
Beet	2 tsp.	yellow	4 hours
Brazil nuts	as needed	red	8 hours
Broccoli	2 Tbsp.	yellow	6 hours
Buckwheat	1 cup	green	8 hours
Chick peas	1 cup	red	12 hours
Clover	2 tsp.	yellow	6 hours
Fenugreek	2 tsp.	yellow	6 hours
Green peas	1 cup	red	8 hours
Lentils	½ cup	green	8 hours
Millet	½ cup	yellow	5 hours
Mung beans	½ cup	green	8 hours
Pea shoots	1 cup	green	8 hours
Pecans	as needed	red	8 hours
Pumpkin	1 cup	red lid	4 hours
Quinoa	½ cup	yellow	3 hours
Sunflower	1 cup	red lid	6 hours
Watermelon	1 cup	green	8 hours
Walnuts	as needed	red	8 hours
Wheatgrass	1 cup	yellow	8 hours

Soaking times for some nuts are included here as well for your reference. After soaking, nuts can be used right away for recipes or for snacks. You may want to dehydrate the nuts prior to eating.

Generally speaking, smaller seeds do not require as much soak time as larger seeds. Because they are physically smaller, seeds like alfalfa, clover, and broccoli have less surface area for the water to penetrate.

Growing Your Own Living Foods

At the end of the soak time drain the water from the sprout vessel. Rinse one time and drain again. Shake any excess water out of your sprouting vessel. Leave your sprouting vessel supported in a position that will allow any excess water to continue to drip drain without cutting off the air supply.

Sprout Vessel	Drain Position
Sprout jar	Leave the jar at a 45 degree angle in a dish rack.
Sprout bag	Hang the bag on a hook above the sink or bowl.
Pitcher method	Sleeve the drilled pitcher inside a regular pitcher.
EasySprouter	Sleeve the inner cup inside the outer cup. Turn the inner cup so that the ribs on the inner cup sit up on the ledge of the outer cup. This creates an air gap between the inner cup and the outer cup. Next, place the small measuring cup on top of the inner cup so that the vent holes are facing up creating a domed lid. This will accelerate sprouting.

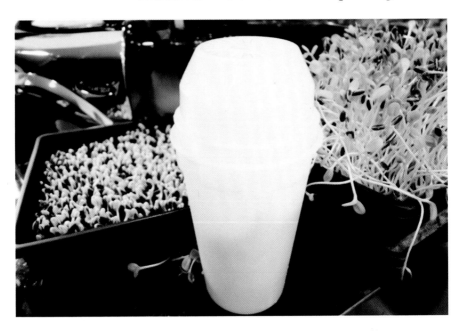

Growing Your Own Living Foods

Rinse with fresh filtered water twice a day for the duration of the rinsing time. This will vary based upon the sprout type.

Seed Type	Rinsing Time	Planting Time*
Adzuki beans	3 days	
Alfalfa	7 days	
Amaranth	1 day	
Beet	7 days	
Broccoli	7 days	
Buckwheat	1 day	12 days
Chick peas	3 days	
Clover	7 days	
Fenugreek	3 days	
Green peas	3 days	
Lentils	3 days	
Millet	1 day	
Mung beans	3 days	
Pea shoots	1 day	7 days
Pumpkin	7 days	
Quinoa	1 day	
Sunflower	1 day	12 days
Watermelon	7 days	
Wheatgrass	1 day	7 days

*Wheatgrass, pea shoots, buckwheat and sunflower require the additional step of planting which is covered in chapters 7 and 8.

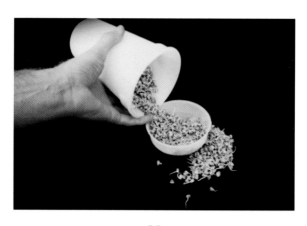

Growing Your Own Living Foods

At the end of the rinsing time your sprouts will be ready to eat! Skip the last rinse to allow your sprouts to dry. What you are not going to use right away can be stored in the refrigerator in a covered container where they will keep for up to five days.

When you are finished with your equipment, clean your lids and jars really, really well with a good, strong organic soap like Seventh Generation dish detergent. You could also use a grapefruit seed extract and water solution. Clean all the threads and all the nooks and crannies.

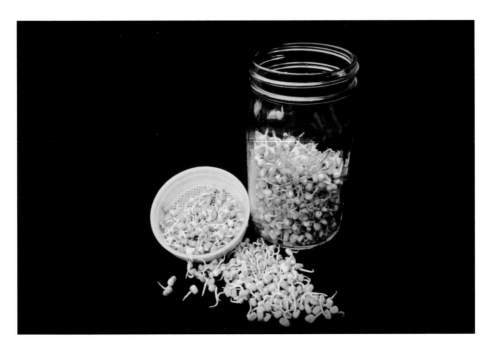

Growing Your Own Living Foods

Chapter 7 – Wheatgrass

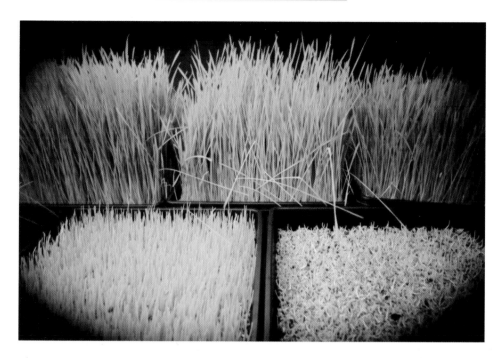

Why Wheatgrass?

Wheatgrass juice is nature's finest medicine. It is a powerful concentrated liquid nutrient. A two ounce shot of wheatgrass juice has the nutritional equivalent of five pounds of the best vegetables. Wheatgrass juice is also a powerful detoxifier pulling poisons, stored toxins, and heavy metals out of the body. It cleans you out from top to bottom, from the inside out!

Wheatgrass juice builds your blood and boosts the immune system. It is a fast-growing, high energy, high frequency plant. Two ounces of wheatgrass juice has the nutritional equivalent of five pounds of the best raw organic vegetables! For example, wheatgrass has twice the amount of Vitamin A as carrots and is higher in Vitamin C than oranges! It contains the full spectrum of B vitamins, as well as calcium, phosphorus, magnesium, sodium and potassium in a balanced ratio. Wheatgrass is a complete source of protein, supplying all of the essential amino acids, and more. It has about 20% of total calories coming from protein. This protein is in the form of poly peptides, simpler and shorter chains of amino acids that the body uses more efficiently in the blood stream and tissues.

In addition to flooding the body with therapeutic dosages of vitamins, minerals, antioxidants, enzymes, and phytonutrients, wheatgrass is also a powerful detoxifier, especially of the liver and blood. It helps neutralize toxins and environmental pollutants in the body. This is because Wheatgrass contains beneficial enzymes that help protect us from carcinogens, including Superoxide Disumates (SOD), that lessens the effects of radiation and digest toxins in the body. It cleanses the body from head to toe of any heavy metals, pollutants and other toxins that may be stored in the body's tissues and organs.

We recommend that you aspire to drink two ounces of wheatgrass juice twice a day. We also use wheatgrass in other therapeutic applications as well. The wheatgrass juice must be consumed fresh - within fifteen minutes of juicing for the best results. The juice should always be taken undiluted and on an empty stomach so the nutrients can be absorbed more efficiently. Powdered and freeze dried wheatgrass supplements are nowhere near as effective as fresh wheatgrass juice. A study was conducted with MIT awhile back comparing frozen and powdered wheatgrass with fresh juiced wheatgrass. The study revealed that frozen and powdered wheatgrass are only two percent as effective as fresh juiced wheatgrass when it is consumed within fifteen minutes. The nutrients quickly begin to oxidize (break down) very quickly after juicing.

When it is consumed fresh it is a living food and has *bio-electricity.* This high vibration energy is literally the life force within the living juice. This resource of life-force energy can potentially unleash powerful renewing vibrations and greater connectivity to one's inner being. These powerful nutrients can also prevent DNA destruction and help protect us from the ongoing effects of pre-mature aging and cellular breakdown. Recent research shows that only *living* foods and juices can restore the electrical charge between the capillaries and the cell walls which boosts the immune system. When it is fresh, wheatgrass juice is the king of living juices.

Growing Your Own Living Foods

Wheatgrass juice is particularly high in chlorophyll among other things. Wheatgrass cleanses and builds the blood due to its high content of chlorophyll. Chlorophyll is the first product of light and therefore contains more healing properties than any other element. All life on this planet comes from the sun. Only green plants can transform the sun's energy into chlorophyll through the process of photosynthesis. . Chlorophyll is known as the 'life-blood' of the plants. This important phytonutrient is what your cells need to heal and to thrive. Drinking wheatgrass juice is like drinking liquid sunshine.

Chlorophyll carries high levels of oxygen (among other things) which is especially powerful in assisting the body to restore abnormalities. The high content of oxygen in chlorophyll helps deliver more oxygen to the blood. We see red blood cell counts rise and blood oxygen levels rise very quickly with the regular drinking of wheatgrass juice and using wheatgrass juice implants. This marker is a key indicator of health recovery for abnormalities, ailments and disease. Oxygen is vital to many body processes, especially for the brain which uses 25% of the oxygen supply. This high oxygen helps support a healthy body.

Growing Your Own Living Foods

How to Grow the Best Wheatgrass

The best type of seed to use for growing wheatgrass is the red hard winter wheat berries. You will also find white wheat, soft wheat, a Spring, Summer, and Fall wheat. None of these will work as well as red hard winter wheat. The first step is to germinate the seeds with water and then to plant the geminated seeds in soil.

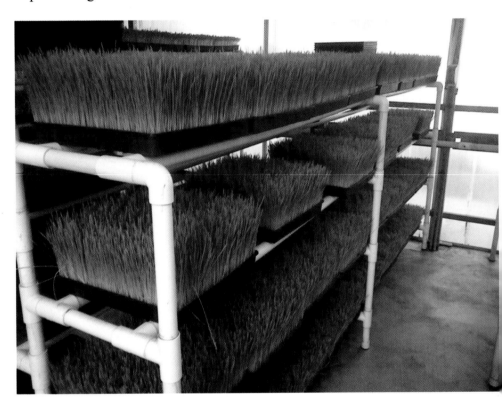

Growing Your Own Living Foods

Mason Jar Method

Here is how to germinate wheatgrass using a Mason jar with a sprouting lid:

1. Place 1 cup of dry seeds in a one quart wide mouth Mason jar. Attach the green sprout lid.

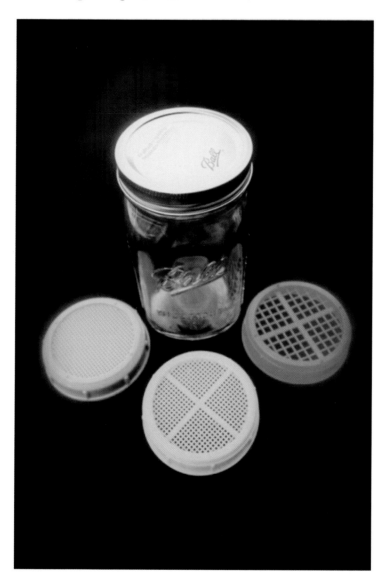

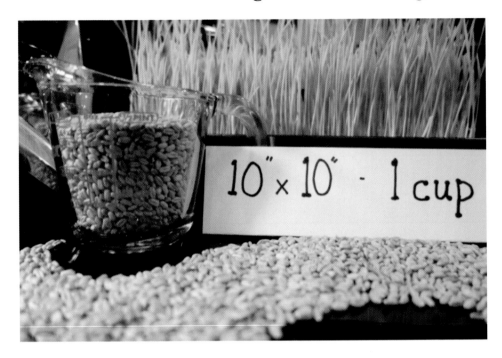

2. Add 3 cups of fresh filtered room temperature water and soak for 8 hours.
3. Drain. Rinse and drain again. Pour the drain water down the sink or use it to water your plants.
4. Place the Mason jar top down at a 45 degree angle in a dish rack to allow any excess water to drain.
5. Over the next 36 hours, rinse three times twelve hours apart using fresh, filtered, room temperature water. Double rinse each time. After each rinse return the jar top down at a 45 degree angle in the dish rack.
6. After the third rinse your sprouts will have a tiny white nub appearing from one end of the seed. That is the "tail" or the root of the plant beginning to emerge. This is the perfect stage for planting. If you continue rinsing the tail will get too long and they will all get tangled together. When you go to spread them out the tails will tear damaging the plant which will reduce your yield.
7. Proceed to the next section entitled "Planting Germinated Wheatgrass Seeds"

Sprout Bag Method

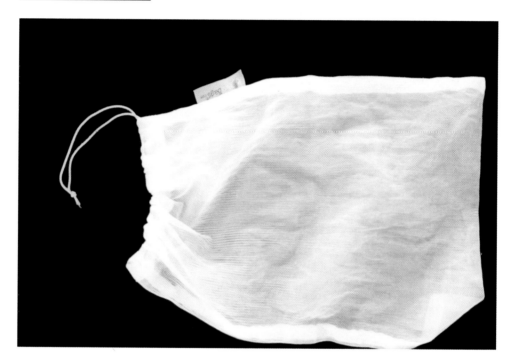

Here is how to grow wheatgrass using a Sprout Bag:

1. Place 1 cup of seeds in a sprout bag.
2. Pull up the drawstrings and submerse the bag in a bowl filled with fresh, filtered room temperature water and soak for 8 hours.
3. Lift the bag from the bowl of water and allow it to drain. Rinse with fresh water and drain again. Pour the drain water down the sink or use it to water your plants.
4. Hang the bag up by the drawstring on a hook above the sink or above a drain pan. If you have one of those tall gooseneck faucets on your sink you can hang your sprout bag up on the neck of your faucet.
5. Rinse three times twelve hours apart using fresh, filtered room temperature water. Double rinse each time.
6. After the third rinse your sprouts will have a tiny white nub appearing from one end of the seed. That is the "tail" or the root of

the plant beginning to emerge. This is the perfect stage for planting. If you continue rinsing the tail will get too long and they will all get tangled together. When you go to spread them out the tails will tear damaging the plant which will reduce your yield.

7. Proceed to the next section entitled "Planting Germinated Wheatgrass Seeds"

Pitcher Method

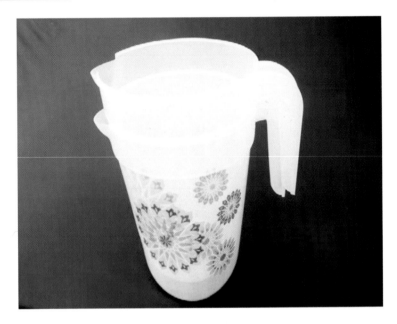

Here is how to grow wheatgrass using the pitcher method:

1. Add 1 cup of seeds to the pitcher with the holes in the bottom.
2. Sleeve the pitcher inside a second unmodified pitcher.
3. Add 3 cups of fresh filtered room temperature water and soak for 8 hours.
4. At the end of the soak time un-sleeve the pitchers to drain the water off. Rinse and drain again.
5. Rinse three times twelve hours apart using fresh, filtered room temperature water. Double rinse each time.

6. After the third rinse your seeds will have a tiny white nub appearing from one end of the seed. That is the "tail" or the root of the plant beginning to emerge. This is the perfect stage for planting. If you continue rinsing the tail will get too long and they will all get tangled together. When you go to spread them out the tails will tear damaging the plant which will reduce your yield.

7. Proceed to the next section entitled "Planting Germinated Wheatgrass Seeds"

EasySprouter Method

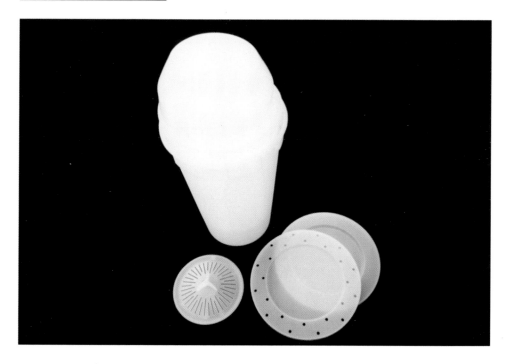

Here is how to grow wheatgrass using the EasySprouter:

1. Sleeve the inner cup inside the outer cup. Index the ribs on the inner cup so they fit inside the keyways of the outer cup. This way, the tops of the two cups will be flush.

2. Place 1 cup of seeds into the inner cup.

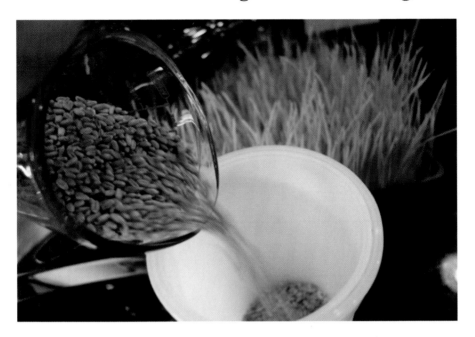

3. Add fresh, filtered, room temperature water up to about an inch from the top and soak for 8 hours.

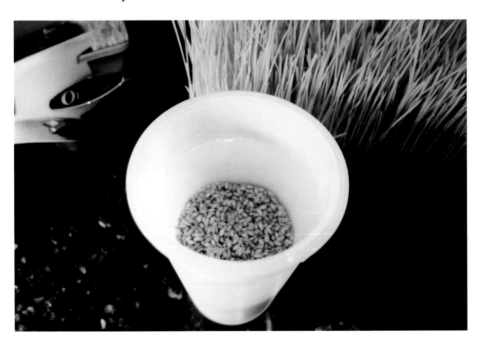

4. At the end of the soak time un-sleeve the inner cup from the outer cup to drain the water. Rinse and drain again. Pour the drain water down the sink or use it to water your plants.

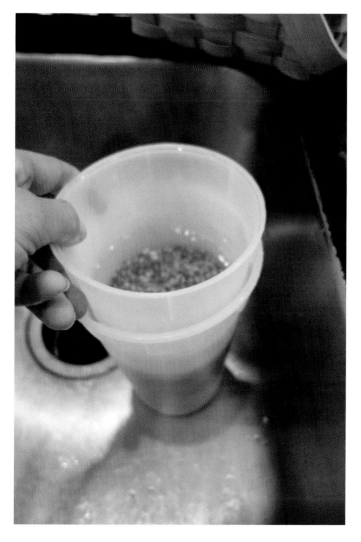

5. Re-sleeve the inner cup back inside the outer cup. Only this time, lift and turn so that the ribs on the inner cup sit up on the ledge of the outer cup. This creates an air gap between the inner cup and the outer cup.

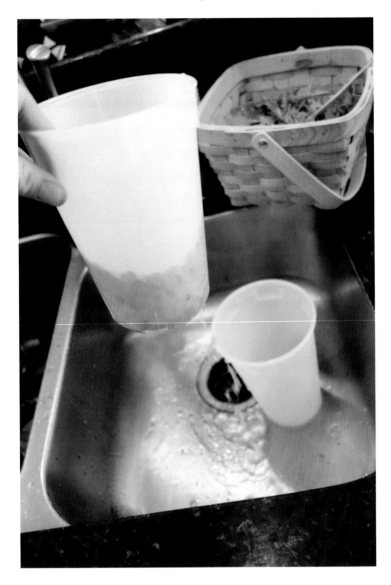

6. Next, place the small measuring cup on top of the inner cup so that the vent holes are facing up creating a domed lid. This creates the "chimney effect."
7. Twelve hours later rinse your seeds using fresh, filtered room temperature water. Reassemble your EasySprouter after each rinse as described in the last two steps.

8. Wait another twelve hours and your seeds will be ready to plant. By now your seeds will have a tiny white nub appearing from one end of the seed. That is the "tail" or the root of the plant beginning to emerge. This is the perfect stage for planting. If you continue rinsing the tail will get too long and they will all get tangled together. When you go to spread them out the tails will tear damaging the plant which will reduce your yield.
9. Proceed to the next section entitled "Planting Germinated Wheatgrass Seeds"

Planting Germinated Wheatgrass Seeds

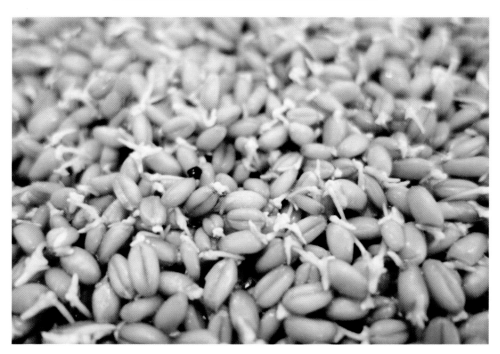

Once the seeds are geminated they are transferred to trays lined with a thin layer of potting mix in the bottom. Make sure your trays have holes in the bottom so they can drain. Support your trays from below so they are not sitting in their own drain water. You could use an inverted Tupperware bin lid sitting your trays on top of some spacers such as extra sprout lids. Or, you could use a multi-tiered rack system with a drain pan all the way on the bottom rung. You can also place a towel underneath the drain pan. Empty your drain pan every couple of days.

1. Using a 10" X 10" square tray, add a thin layer of 100% organic potting mix. Spread the potting mix out evenly in the tray breaking up any clumps and picking out any sticks or rocks.

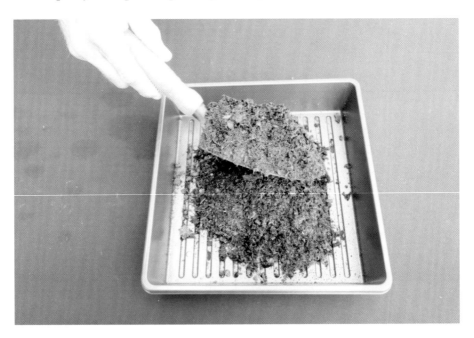

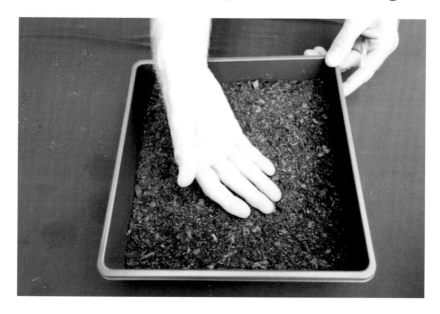

2. Take a second empty tray and place it on top of the potting mix.
    Using the palms of both hands press down firmly to compact the
    potting mix. The depth should be about ½ inch thick after
    compression. Adjust the amount of potting mix and re-compress as
    necessary.

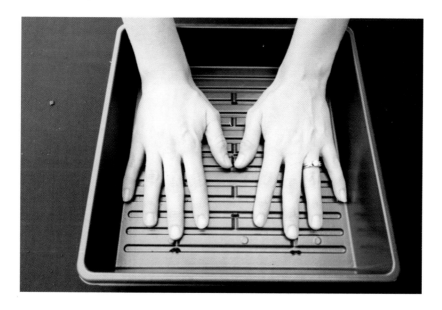

3. Using a misting bottle filled with fresh filtered water, pre-moisten the surface of the potting mix by spraying it heavily. You do not have to get the tray dripping at this point. Just make sure the surface of the potting mix is well moistened.

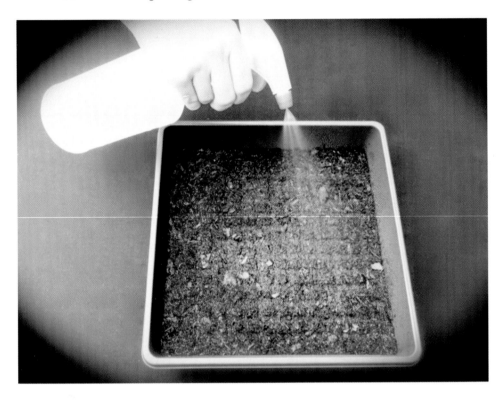

4. Spread your geminated seeds out evenly on top of the moistened potting mix. Your 1 cup of dry seeds that you started out with will now have swollen to about 1.5 cups. This is the perfect amount for a 10" X 10" tray. Lightly brush the germinated seeds out across the surface of the potting mix. You are not pressing them down into the potting mix and you are not going to cover the seeds with any soil. It should be just a single layer thick and just touching side by side. No seeds should be piled on top of each other. If you get this right you should not see any gaps in the soil.

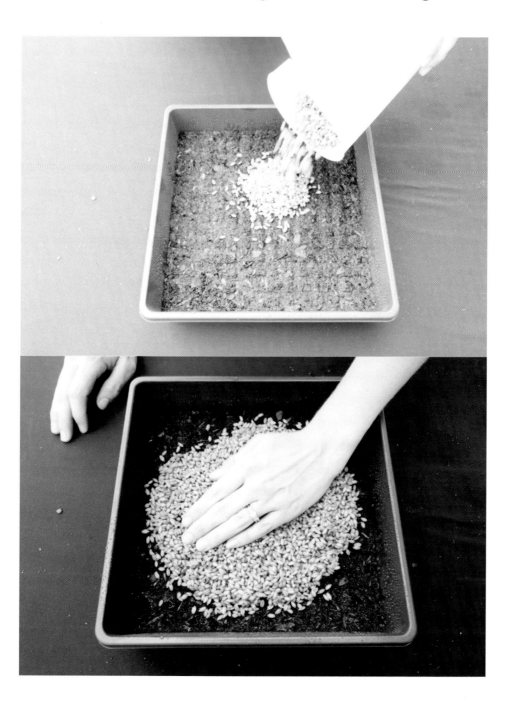

5. Using your misting bottle mist your planted geminated seeds heavy.

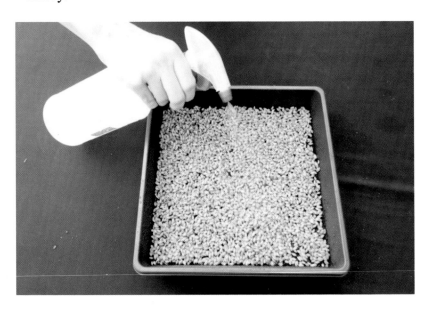

6. Cover with a second empty tray. The purpose of the cover tray is to keep your roots from drying out too quickly.

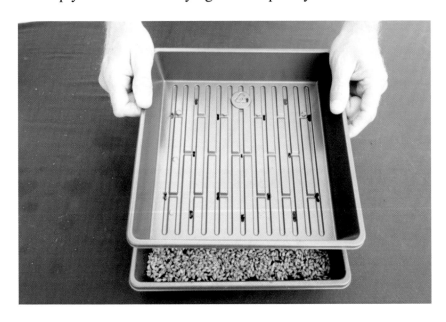

7. Water twice a day for seven or eight days. Water it heavy each time until the tray just starts to drip. Keep your tray propped up using spacers so it is not sitting in its' own drain water. You can also use a multi-tiered ventilated rack for proper drainage.

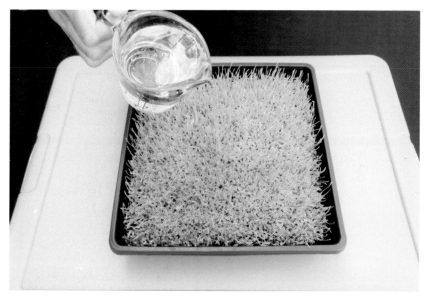

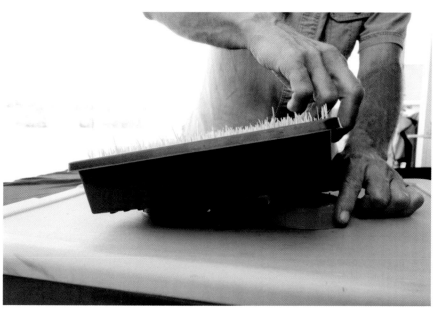

8. Replace the cover tray after each watering for the first three days. The cover tray is not needed after day three. By day four the roots will have figured out which way is "up" and will be long enough to find their way into the bottom of the tray and be protected by the moisture in the potting mix.

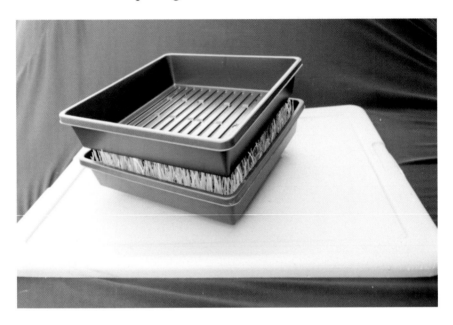

9. Harvest your sprouts at the beginning of the jointing stage or sooner. This usually takes about seven days for wheatgrass.

Growing Your Own Living Foods

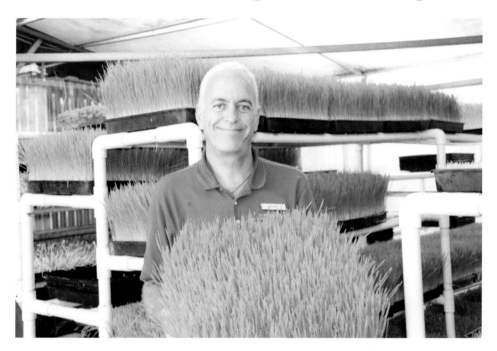

A 10" X 10" tray will yield up to one pound of wheatgrass. This will produce up to nine ounces of wheatgrass juice when using a good quality auger style juicer. What you are not going to use right away you can store them dry in the refrigerator in a covered container where they will keep for up to five days. But, fresh is best so I recommend growing in smaller trays so you have less wheatgrass stored in the refrigerator for a shorter period of time.

When you are finished with your equipment, clean your jars, lids and trays jars really, really well with a good strong natural organic soap like Seventh Generation dish detergent. You could also use grape fruit seed extract and water solution. Clean in all the threads, ribs, corners and in all the nooks and crannies. Wheatgrass is very high in protein and high in enzymes. You don't want to transfer any proteins or enzymes from one batch to the next. This could lead to mold.

Growing Your Own Living Foods

Wheatgrass Juice Taste

Not all wheatgrass juice will taste the same. The difference in taste will vary depending upon how you grow it. In order to grow the sweetest tasting wheatgrass you will need to observe three rules:

1. Harvest the entire tray at the beginning of the jointing stage, or sooner. The jointing stage is a botanical term for when the grass is graduating from a baby to an adult. This is when the grass is the sweetest, the most tender and the most nutritious. The older it gets the more bitter it gets. Kind of like us☺! But, every day the wheatgrass grows past the jointing stage it ages 40 years!
2. Lighting. You need plenty of indirect sunlight and plenty of artificial light to supplement for cloudy days. But, no direct sunlight, ever. If you grow in direct sunlight your grass will be more bitter.
3. Freshness. Your cut wheatgrass will last in the refrigerator for up to five days but, fresh is always best.

Loving Intentions

Grow your wheatgrass with lots of loving intention☺! Convey plenty of your positive energy to your wheatgrass as it moves through the growing process. Think positive thoughts and speak loving words of gratitude to your grass as it is growing for the healing medicine and life-force energy it will convey to you. Play soft, classical music to your plants during daylight hours.

Soil vs. Hydroponic

We recommend growing tray sprouts in soil as opposed to growing hydroponically. Growing in soil serves two functions. First, the soil acts as a moisture manager so you do not have to water as often. Second, organic soil will add some nutrients to the sprouts. Growing hydroponically takes more time since you have to water more often and costs money since you need to purchase a non-reusable growth media such as growing blankets. You should also use a natural liquid fertilizer such as Ocean Solution when growing hydroponically.

Growing Your Own Living Foods

The best type of soil to use is an organic potting mix. This is also known as a "seed starting mix" which it is available in bags at any nursery or garden center. It may also be available in bulk at larger nurseries and garden supply centers. You can also make your own potting mix by blending 50% peat moss or coconut husk shavings, 25% vermiculite and 25% pearlite.

The primary objective of the potting mix is to provide an equal distribution of moisture while allowing adequate drainage. Avoid using potting soil, topsoil or compost. These are different products and will not allow enough drainage which could lead to mold.

Yield

Depending upon the type of juicer you are using a 10" X 10" tray will yield up to 9 ounces of juice which is enough for two people for one day. That is if you each intend to drink two ounces twice a day. I like the easy to clean Omega juicer. Plant a new tray and harvest a completed tray every day. This way you will always have seven trays of wheatgrass growing in various stages. You can use the small Hydrosol rack which has seven shelves – one for each day of the week. The Hippocrates store can provide you with the Hydrosol racks, trays, seeds, and sprout lids and they will ship worldwide. Or, you can use any type of commercially available rack storage or you can build your own.

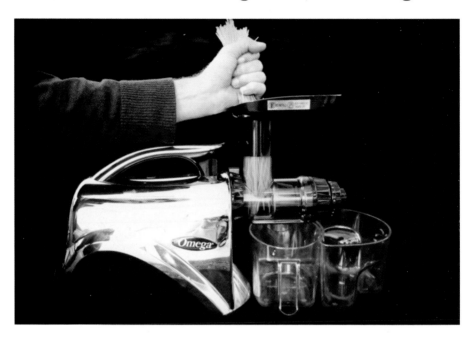

Chapter 8 –Pea, Buckwheat, and Sunflower Sprouts

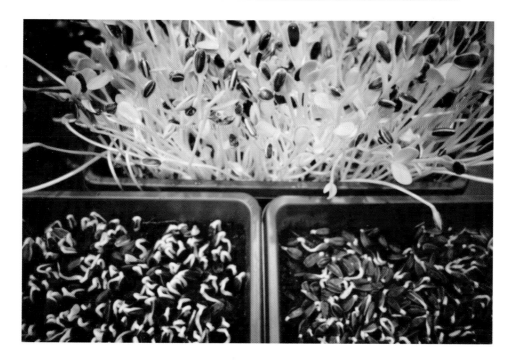

Pea Sprouts

You grow pea sprouts exactly the same way as wheatgrass. For seeds you can use green peas, speckled peas or brown peas. Just make sure they are whole, organic and raw. Split peas, frozen peas, or peas that have been heat processed in any way or irradiated will not work. The best type of seed to use is "pea shoots." This type of pea will grow the fastest and the tallest. See Chapter 7 and follow the instructions just like you are growing wheatgrass.

Buckwheat Sprouts

You grow buckwheat sprouts exactly the same way as wheatgrass and peas sprouts except it takes twelve days to grow instead of seven. When you buy buckwheat you can get them "hulled" which means the seeds have been removed from the shell or "un-hulled" which means the seeds are still in the shell. Hulled buckwheat will be ivory in color. After soaking, hulled buckwheat seeds are typically used for making buckwheat groats as a breakfast cereal or added to flax seeds to make dehydrated crackers. However, when you want to make the tall green leafy buckwheat sprout greens you must use un-hulled seeds which will be brown in color. Always be sure the seeds are whole, organic, raw and commercially distributed with the intention of sprouting. See Chapter 7 and follow the instructions just like you are growing wheatgrass.

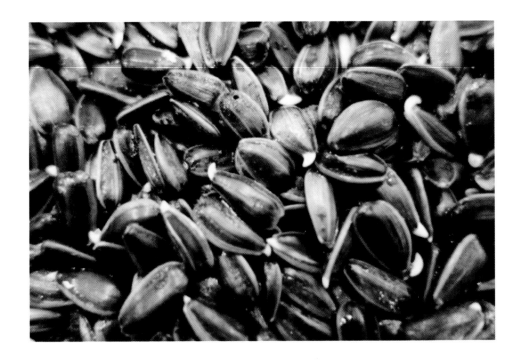

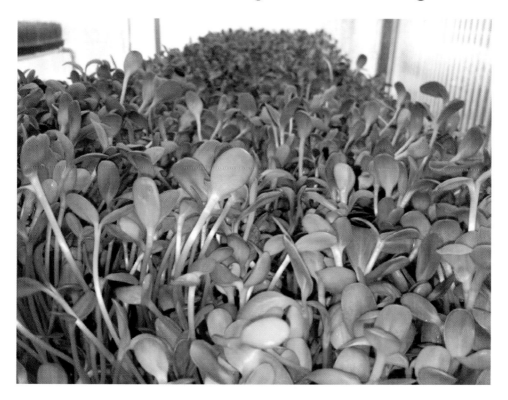

How to Grow the Best Sunflower Sprouts

Just like buckwheat seeds, sunflower seeds are available hulled (which will appear ivory in color) or un-hulled (which will appear black or black with a white stripe.) After soaking, hulled sunflower seeds are typically dehydrated and used for snacking or used in recipes. However, when you want to make the tall green leafy sunflower sprout greens you must use un-hulled seeds. Always be sure the seeds are whole, organic, raw and commercially distributed with the intention of sprouting.

One of the secrets to successfully growing sunflower sprouts is to develop strong and vertical stalks. This can be done in two stages by first growing under pressure for five days and then, by growing in the dark for an additional three days.

Growing Your Own Living Foods

Growing under pressure for the first five days accomplishes two things. First, by using the force of gravity it tells your budding sunflower seeds which way to grow. That is, which way is up. Second, it is like sending your sunflower sprouts to the gym. They have to lift weights so, they develop strong stalks. The first step is to germinate the seeds with water and then to plant the geminated seeds in soil.

Growing in the dark with an empty domed cover tray for an additional three days also helps to keep your sunfower stems growing vertically because the sunflower wants to get to the light. So, it keeps growing "up."

Mason Jar Method

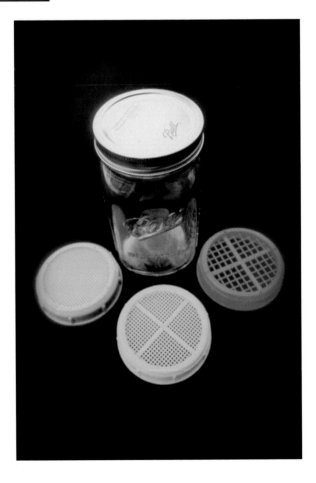

Growing Your Own Living Foods

Here is how to germinate sunflower seeds using a Mason jar with a sprouting lid:

1. Place 1 cup of seeds in a one quart wide mouth Mason jar. Attach the green sprout lid.

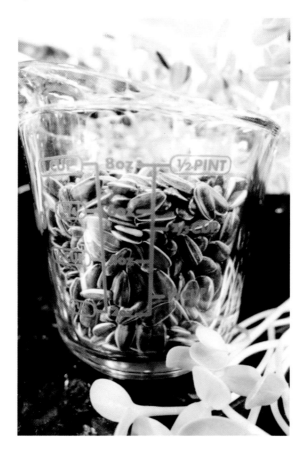

2. Add 3 cups of fresh filtered room temperature water and soak for 8 hours.
3. You will notice the sunflower seeds will float to the top of the water which means that you will need to stir a few times during the first hour to make sure all the seeds get covered with water.
4. Drain. Rinse and drain again. Pour the drain water down the sink or use it to water your plants.

5. Place the Mason jar top down at a 45 degree angle in a dish rack to allow any excess water to drain.
6. Over the next 36 hours, rinse three times twelve hours apart using fresh, filtered, room temperature water. Double rinse each time. After each rinse return the jar top down at a 45 degree angle in the dish rack.
7. After the third rinse your sprouts will have a tiny white nub appearing from one end of the seed. That is the "tail" or the root of the plant beginning to emerge. This is the perfect stage for planting. If you continue rinsing beyond 36 hours the tail will get too long and they will all get tangled together. When you go to spread them out the tails will tear damaging the plant which will reduce your yield.
8. Proceed to the next section entitled "Planting Germinated Sunflower Seeds"

Growing Your Own Living Foods

Sprout Bag Method

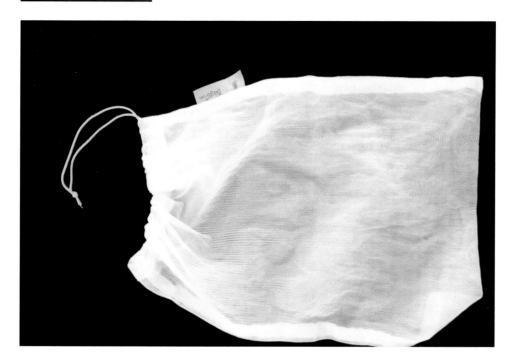

Here is how to germinate sunflower seeds using a Sprout Bag:

1. Place 1 cup of seeds in a sprout bag.
2. Pull up the drawstrings and submerse the bag in a bowl filled with fresh, filtered room temperature water and soak for 8 hours.
3. You will notice the sunflower seeds will float to the top of the water which means that you will need to push the bag below the water line a few times during the first hour to make sure all the seeds get covered with water.
4. After 8 hours lift the bag from the bowl of water and allow it to drain. Rinse with fresh water and drain again. Pour the drain water down the sink or use it to water your plants.
5. Hang the bag up by the drawstring on a hook above the sink or above a drain pan. If you have one of those tall gooseneck faucets on your sink you can hang your sprout bag up on the neck of your faucet.

6. Over the next 36 hours rinse three times twelve hours apart using fresh, filtered room temperature water. Double rinse each time.

7. After the third rinse your sprouts will have a tiny white nub appearing from one end of the seed. That is the "tail" or the root of the plant beginning to emerge. This is the perfect stage for planting. If you continue rinsing beyond 36 hours the tail will get too long and they will all get tangled together. When you go to spread them out the tails will tear damaging the plant which will reduce your yield.

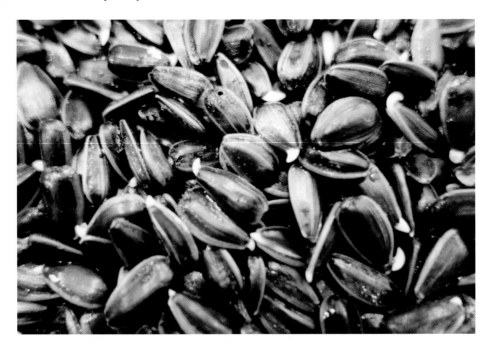

8. Proceed to the next section entitled "Planting Germinated Sunflower Seeds"

Growing Your Own Living Foods

Pitcher Method

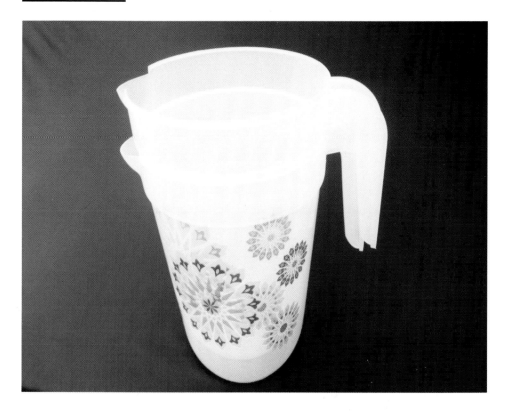

Here is how to germinate sunflower seeds using the pitcher method:

1. Add 1 cup of seeds to the pitcher with the holes in the bottom.
2. Sleeve the pitcher inside a second unmodified pitcher.
3. Add 3 cups of fresh filtered room temperature water and soak for 8 hours.
4. You will notice the sunflower seeds will float to the top of the water which means that you will need to push the bag below the water line a few times during the first hour to make sure all the seeds get covered with water.
5. At the end of the soak time un-sleeve the pitchers to drain the water off. Rinse and drain again.
6. Over the next 36 hours rinse three times twelve hours apart using fresh, filtered room temperature water. Double rinse each time.

7. After the third rinse your sprouts will have a tiny white nub appearing from one end of the seed. That is the "tail" or the root of the plant beginning to emerge. This is the perfect stage for planting. If you continue rinsing beyond 36 hours the tail will get too long and they will all get tangled together. When you go to spread them out the tails will tear damaging the plant which will reduce your yield.
8. Proceed to the next section entitled "Planting Germinated Sunflower Seeds"

EasySprouter Method

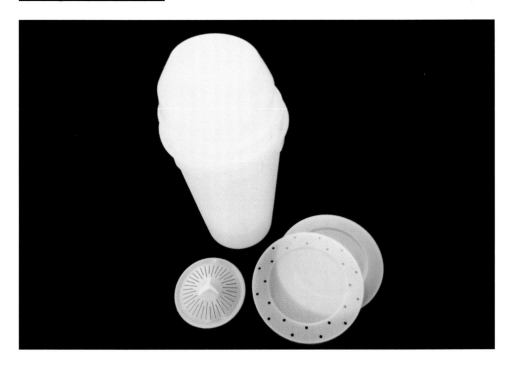

Here is how to grow wheatgrass using the EasySprouter:

1. Sleeve the inner cup inside the outer cup. Index the ribs on the inner cup so they fit inside the keyways of the outer cup. This way, the tops of the two cups will be flush.
2. Place 1 cup of seeds into the inner cup.

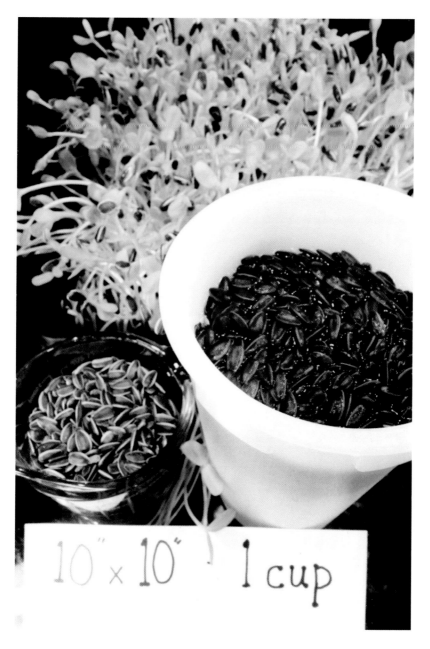

3. Add fresh, filtered, room temperature water up to about an inch
   from the top and soak for 8 hours.

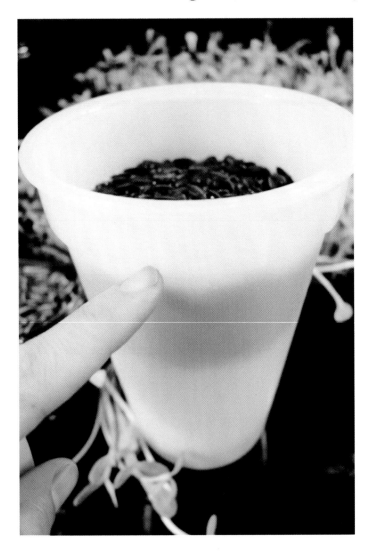

4. You will notice the sunflower seeds will float to the top of the water which means that you will need to stir a few times during the first hour to make sure all the seeds get covered with water. In the case of the EasySprouter there is a trick. You can take the domed lid and install it upside down to push the floating seeds below the level of the water and then install one of the lids to keep the domed lid down. This way you do not need to keep coming back and stirring during the first hour.

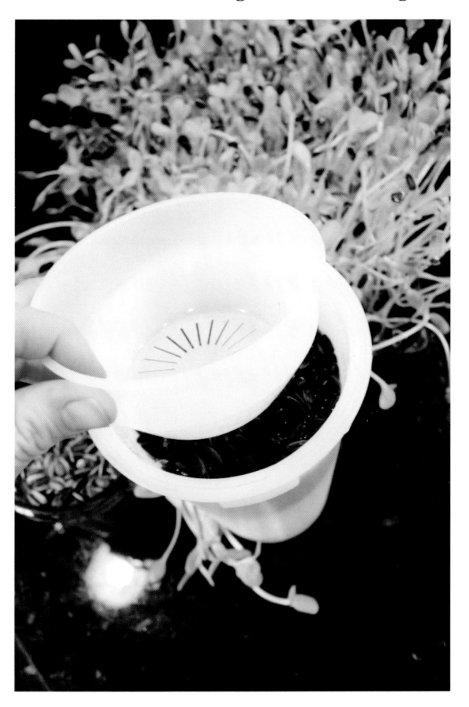

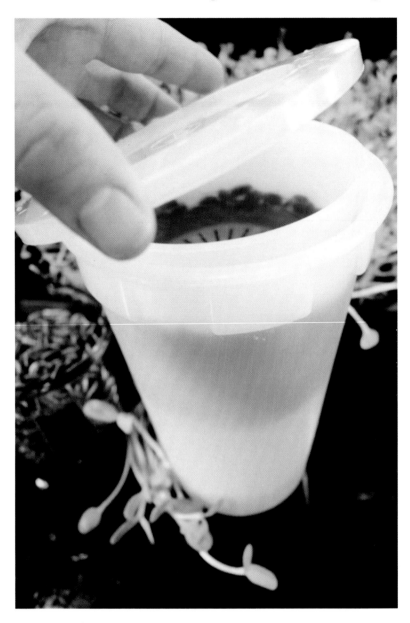

5. At the end of the soak time un-sleeve the inner cup from the outer cup to drain the water. Rinse and drain again. Pour the drain water down the sink or use it to water your plants.

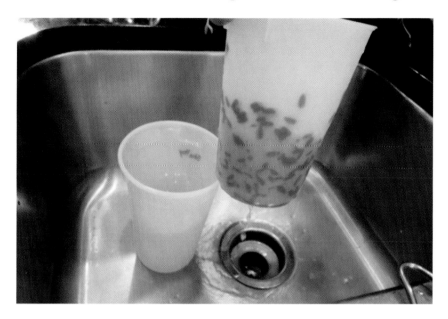

6. Re-sleeve the inner cup back inside the outer cup. Only this time, lift and turn so that the ribs on the inner cup sit up on the ledge of the outer cup. This creates an air gap between the inner cup and the outer cup.

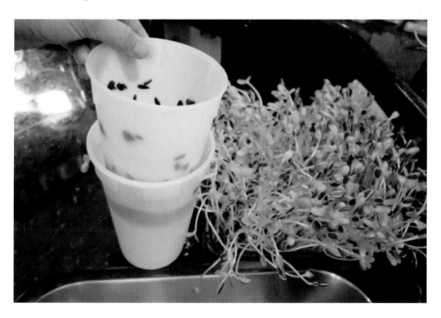

7. Next, place the small measuring cup on top of the inner cup so that the vent holes are facing up creating a domed lid. This creates the "chimney effect."

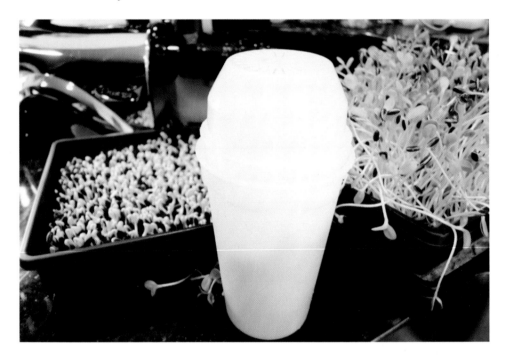

8. Twelve hours later rinse your seeds using fresh, filtered room temperature water. Reassemble your EasySprouter after each rinse as described in the last two steps.
9. Wait another twelve hours and your seeds will be ready to plant. By now your seeds will have a tiny white nub appearing from one end of the seed. That is the "tail" or the root of the plant beginning to emerge. This is the perfect stage for planting. If you continue rinsing the tail will get too long and they will all get tangled together. When you go to spread them out the tails will tear damaging the plant which will reduce your yield.
10. Proceed to the next section entitled "Planting Germinated Sunflower Seeds"

Growing Your Own Living Foods

Planting Germinated Sunflower Seeds

Once the seeds are geminated they are transferred to trays lined with a thin layer of potting mix in the bottom. Make sure your trays have holes in the bottom so they can drain. Support your trays from below so they are not sitting in their own drain water. You could use an inverted Tupperware bin lid sitting your trays on top of some spacers such as extra sprout lids. Or, you could use a multi-tiered rack system with a drain pan all the way on the bottom rung. You can also place a towel underneath the drain pan. Empty your drain pan every couple of days.

1. Using a 10" X 10" square tray, add a thin layer of 100% organic potting mix. Spread the potting mix out evenly in the tray breaking up any clumps and picking out any sticks or rocks.

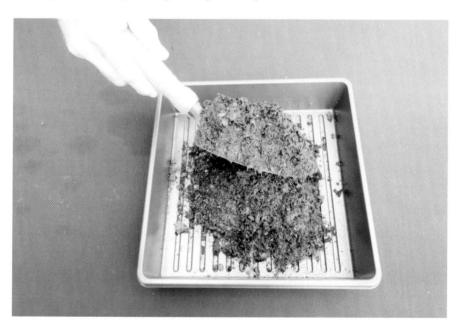

2. Take a second empty tray and place it on top of the potting mix. Using the palms of both hands press down firmly to compact the potting mix. The depth should be about 1 inch thick after compression. Adjust the amount of potting mix to obtain the desired depth and re-compress as necessary.

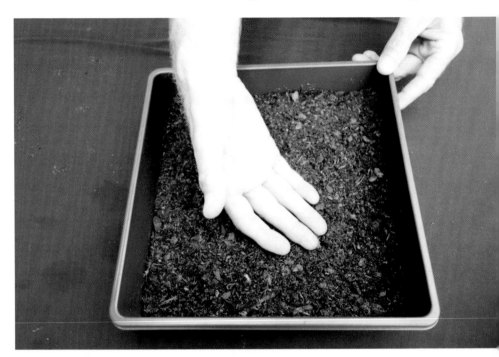

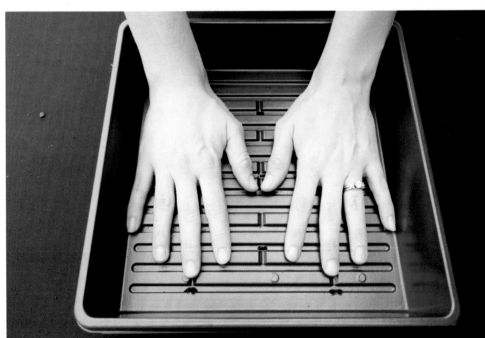

3. Using a misting bottle filled with fresh filtered water, pre-moisten the surface of the potting mix by spraying it heavily. You do not have to get the tray dripping at this point. Just make sure the surface of the potting mix is well moistened.

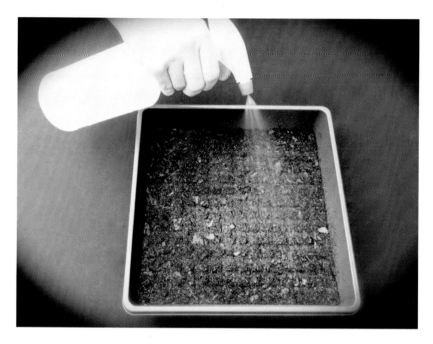

4. Spread your geminated seeds out evenly on top of the moistened potting mix. Your 1 cup of dry seeds that you started out with will now have swollen to about 1.5 cups. This is the perfect amount for a 10" X 10" tray. Lightly brush the germinated seeds out across the surface of the potting mix. You are not pressing them down into the potting mix and you are not going to cover the seeds with any soil. It should be just a single layer thick and just touching side by side. No seeds should be piled on top of each other. If you get this right you should not see any gaps in the soil.

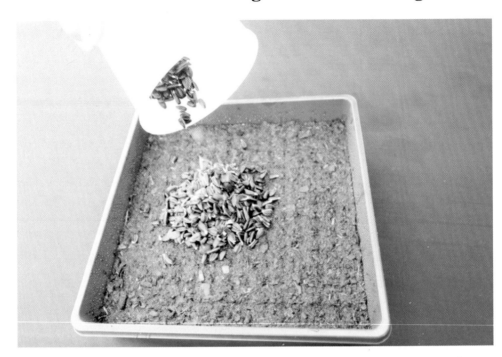

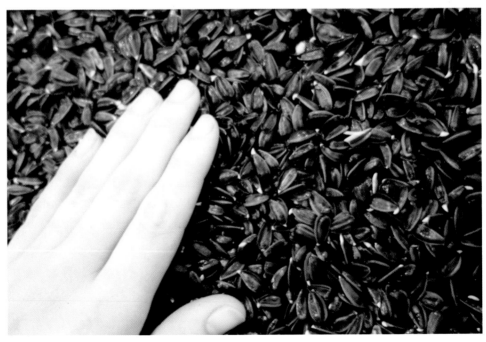

5. Using your misting bottle mist your geminated and planted seeds heavy.

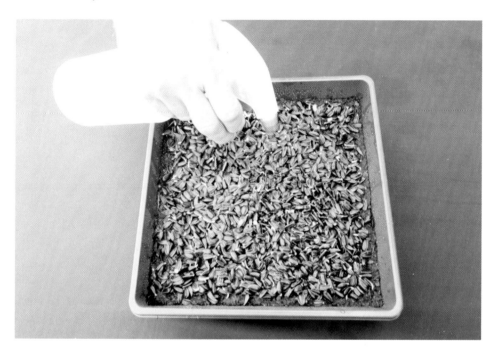

6. Cover your sunflower tray with a weighted tray. Your weighted tray can be filled with dirt, bricks, books, rocks or concrete. The purpose of the weighted tray is to keep your roots from drying out too quickly and to develop strong and vertical sunflower stalks.

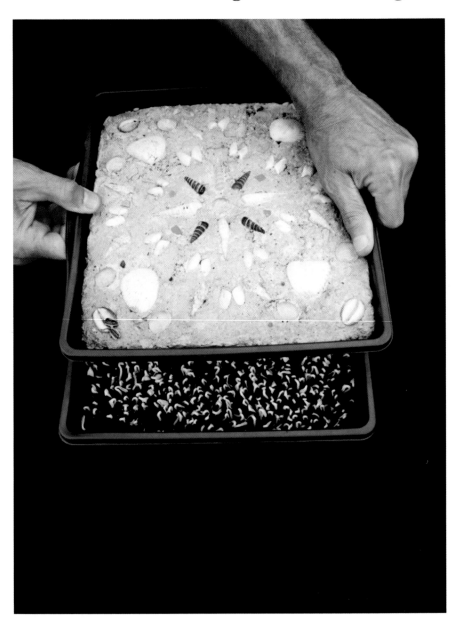

7. Water twice a day for a total of twelve to fourteen days. Water heavy each time until the tray just starts to drip. Keep your tray propped up using spacers so it is not sitting in its' own drain water. You can also use a multi-tiered ventilated rack for proper drainage.

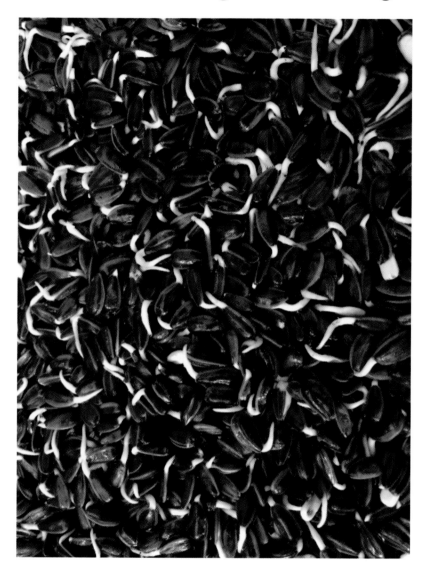

8. Return the weighted tray on top of your growing sprouts after each watering for the first five days. By the end of day five you should see a gap between the bottom tray and the weighted top tray. When you see this gap you do not need the weighted tray any more. Replace the weighted tray with an empty tray that is turned upside down to create a "domed lid." The domed lid also helps to develop vertical sunflower stalks.

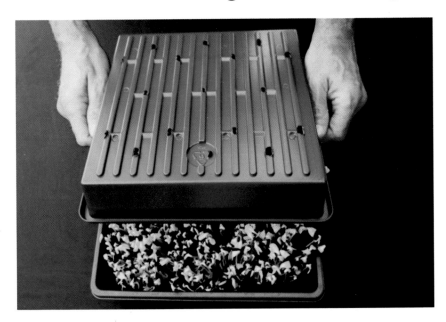

9. Keep watering twice a day returning the "domed lid" on top of your growing sprouts after each watering. When you see a gap between the bottom tray and the "domed lid" then, you do not need the cover any more.

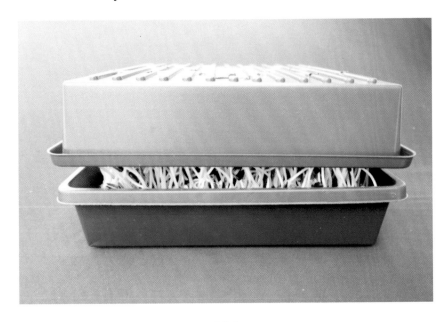

10. Your sprouts are ready to harvest at the beginning of the jointing stage or sooner. The jointing stage is when you see a second growth begin to emerge from between the two primary "water leaves." This usually takes about twelve to fourteen days for sunflower sprouts. This is when your sprouts are the sweetest, the most nutritious, and the most tender.

11. Harvest the entire tray all at once to halt the growing process. Using a knife or a pair of scissors grab a clump of sprouts one at a time and cut as close to the soil line as possible. Discard any brown stem pieces. What you are not going to use right away you can store dry in the refrigerator where they will keep for up to five days. Rinse your sprouts using cool water prior to use.

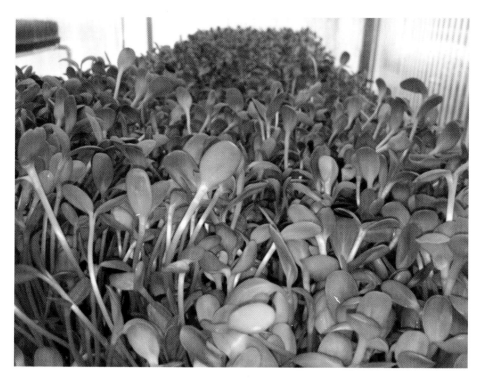

12. When you are finished with your equipment, clean your jars, lids and trays jars really, really well with a good strong natural organic soap like Seventh Generation dish detergent. You could also use grape fruit seed extract and water solution. Clean in all the threads,

ribs, corners and in all the nooks and crannies. Sprouts are very high in protein and high in enzymes. You don't want to transfer any proteins or enzymes from one batch to the next as this could lead to mold.

Yield

A 10" X 10" tray will yield up to 28 ounces of sunflower sprouts. This will produce up to 21 ounces of sunflower sprout juice when using a good quality auger style juicer. What you are not going to use right away you can store them dry in the refrigerator in a covered container where they will keep for up to five days. But, fresh is best so I recommend growing in smaller trays so you have less sunflower sprouts stored in the refrigerator for a shorter period of time.

Removing the Hulls

The secret to removing the hulls is in the type of seeds. The white stripe seeds which are a little less expensive and are easier to find, will shed about 50% of their hulls during the growing process. The back oil seeds which are a little smaller and a little harder to find, will shed about 99% of their hulls all by themselves during the growing process.

Any remaining hulls can be removed during harvesting by cutting a handful at a time from the root mat. While holding them firmly in your hand swiftly swing your arm down and back while snapping your wrist like you are cracking a whip. This will shake most of the remaining hulls off. The last few will have to hand-picked off from the tip of the sprouts.

Loving Intentions

Grow all your sprouts with lots of loving intention☺! Convey plenty of your positive energy to your sprouts as they move through the growing process. Think positive thoughts and speak loving words of gratitude to your grass as it is growing for the healing medicine and life-force energy it will convey to you. Play soft, classical music to your plants during daylight hours.

Growing Your Own Living Foods

Soil vs. Hydroponic

We recommend growing tray sprouts in soil as opposed to growing hydroponically. Growing in soil serves two functions. First, the soil acts as a moisture manager so you do not have to water as often. Second, organic soil will add some nutrients to the sprouts. Growing hydroponically takes more time since you have to water more often and costs money since you need to purchase a non-reusable growth media such as growing blankets. You should also use a natural liquid fertilizer such as Ocean Solution when growing hydroponically.

The best type of soil to use is an organic potting mix. This is also known as a "seed starting mix" which it is available in bags at any nursery or garden center. It may also be available in bulk at larger nurseries and garden supply centers. You can also make your own potting mix by blending 50% peat moss or coconut husk shavings, 25% vermiculite and 25% pearlite.

The primary objective of the potting mix is to provide an equal distribution of moisture while allowing adequate drainage. Avoid using potting soil, topsoil or compost. These are different products and will not allow enough drainage which could lead to mold.

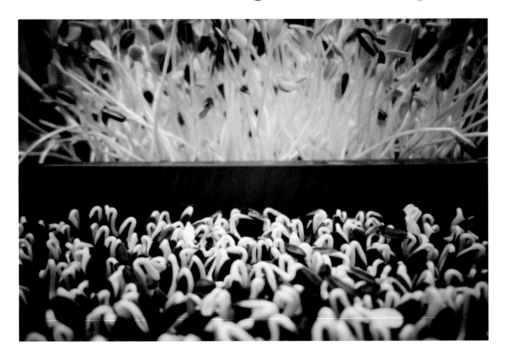

Chapter 9 – Specialty Sprouts

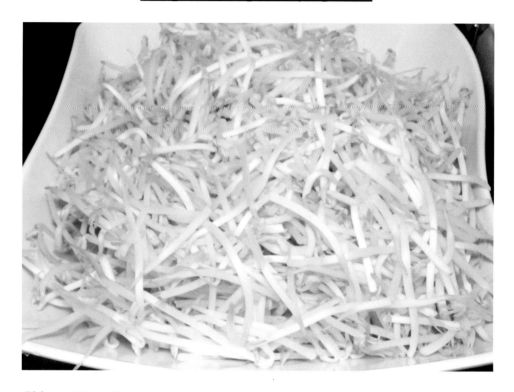

Chinese Bean Sprouts

Typically you will find these types of sprouts in a Chinese restaurant in a stir fry. Only, we don't want you to stir fry anything here☺! You start with the same mung bean seed that we used to grow the regular green mung bean sprout. The difference between the thick-rooted Chinese bean sprout and the green mung bean sprout is not in the seed. The difference is in the process. In order to grow the thick-rooted Chinese bean sprout you have to grow them under pressure - a *lot* of pressure.

This is where the stackable pitcher method comes in handy because you can sleeve a third weighted pitcher right on top of your growing sprouts. This weighted pitcher has to be really heavy. It should be at least ten pounds. For weight you can simply fill a third pitcher with water, rocks, dirt, or concrete.

Growing Your Own Living Foods

You will also be soaking and rinsing using lukewarm water which is about 100 degrees. This is as opposed to room temperature water which is about 75 degrees. Lukewarm water is about the same as your body temperature. So, when you put your hand in lukewarm water it should not feel cool and it should not feel hot. It should feel about like your body temperature. Using the warmer water makes your sprouts grow faster.

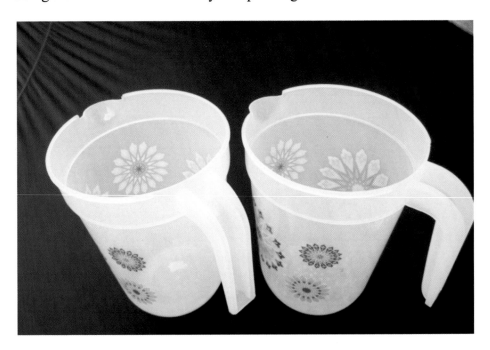

Here is how to grow the thick-rooted Chinese bean sprouts using the weighted pitcher method:

1. Pour the mung bean seeds (½ cup for a 2 quart pitcher or 1 cup for a 4 quart pitcher) into the pitcher with the holes in the bottom.
2. Sleeve this pitcher inside a second unmodified pitcher.
3. Add at least 2 cups of fresh, filtered, lukewarm water and soak for 8 hours.
4. Un-sleeve the pitchers to drain the water off. Rinse and drain again.
5. Rinse twice a day for five days using fresh, filtered, lukewarm water. Double rinse each time.

6. Your sprouts are finished when the tails or the roots of your sprouts are about 1-2 inches long.
7. Enjoy!

Yields approximately five cups (for a 2 quart pitcher or, ten cups for a 4 quart pitcher) in five days. Sprouts you are not going to use right away can be dried and stored in the refrigerator in a covered container where they will keep for up to two days.

When you are finished with your pitchers clean them really, really well with a good strong organic soap like Seventh Generation dish detergent. You could also use grapefruit seed extract and water solution. Clean in all the corners and in all the nooks and crannies.

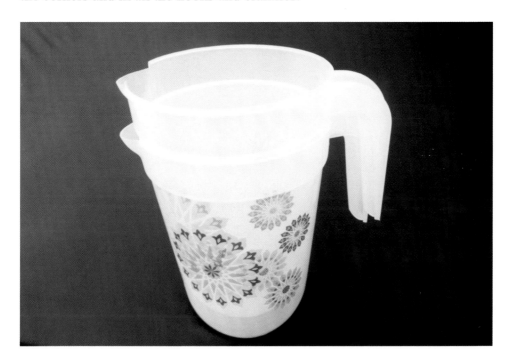

<u>Chia and Flax Sprouts</u>

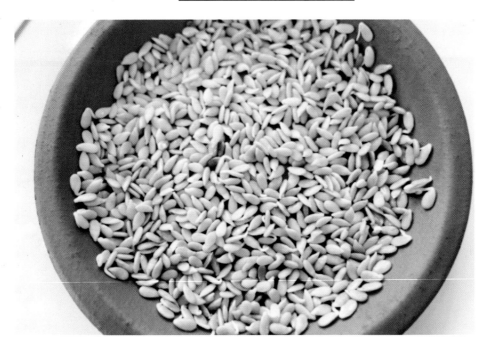

Chia and flax are known as the mucilaginous sprouts. This is because of the "sticky" protein gel that is produced when the seeds get wet. Unlike other sprouts the seeds are not soaked first. Instead, we soak the sprouting vessel which is this case is an unglazed terra-cotta saucer.

Growth Process:
1. Soak an 8" unglazed terra-cotta saucer in water for 2 hours.
2. Drain the saucer and sprinkle 1 teaspoon of whole seeds evenly in the saucer. Try to leave some space between the seeds.
3. Mist lightly and cover with a second saucer.
4. Mist twice a day for seven days. You don't need the cover saucer after day three.
5. Keep in a brightly lit area from day four through seven.

Maturity Time:
- Seven days

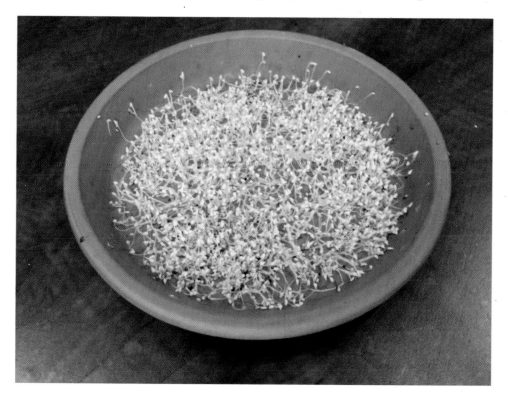

<u>Chapter 10 – Eating Healthy in the Real World</u>

In today's busy world it can seem very difficult to maintain a healthy lifestyle. However, there are a few tricks that can help you incorporate healthy eating into your every-changing daily schedule.

Luck favors the prepared. Set yourself up for success!

Motivation is the key – discover your life's passion and pursue it! You must realize that you are needed, wanted, and desired on this planet. Each one of you is unique and you have a special purpose to achieve in this life. You can call it a spiritual goal. Nobody else can fulfill your unique mission.

You must discover your life's purpose and pursue it with passion! You may want to consider a life coach to help you find your life's passion. I believe most people already know deep down on some level how to eat properly. You simply must believe you are worth it!

Educate Yourself -
Take raw food "cooking" classes to increase your meal plan.
Read raw food books and articles on the internet.
Attend raw food teaching lectures.

Immerse yourself in the healthy eating world -
Attend raw food dinners and offer to host raw potlucks at your home.
Visit Raw Food social websites like giveittomeraw.com.

Go slowly! 10% each month. Set your ultimate goal for 80% raw 100% vegan.

Success at Home!

1. Set up your kitchen equipment – blender, juicer, food processer, dehydrator. If you cannot afford them right away ask for Christmas and Birthday gifts. Learn how to use them.

2. Stock up your pantry and fridge – with plenty of fruits, veggies, nuts, seeds, superfoods, WildBars and BGBars.
3. Green Smoothies are your secret weapon – learn how to make several delicious versions. Make two quarts for breakfast every morning.
4. Be a living example for your friends and loved ones. Try not to preach. They will notice your improved looks, attitude and energy!
5. Grow your own sprouts! It is economical and fun! Kids love to get involved in sprouting.
6. Don't introduce raw foods to your family with wheatgrass juice and energy soup. Go to raw food cooking classes and learn how to make raw food delicious and attractive!

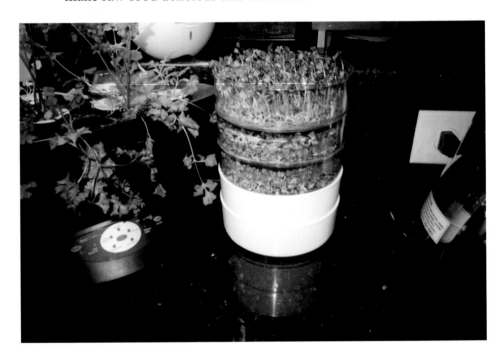

Success Going Out to Restaurants!

If you have time to sit down to eat, an independent restaurant is always more flexible with how you place your order. A chain eatery is not usually set up to handle requests to omit meats or add more veggies. In fact, the nicer the restaurant, the more they will go out of their way to please the customer. Even though they have vegetarian options, try to avoid buffet-style restaurants, as they are loaded with unhealthy, starchy fattening, and fried foods.

If you don't see something you like on the menu of an independent restaurant, ask the waiter to see if the chef will prepare a special vegetarian dish of his own. Quite often they will enjoy creating something out of the ordinary. Be sure to send your praises back via the server to pave the way for the rest of us!

Surprisingly, you can eat very healthfully even at a steak house. How can that be? you wonder, since the main goal is not to eat meat. It's possible because the best side dishes for a steak are beautiful salads, baked potatoes, and vegetables. Just ask them to hold the cheese!

Italian restaurants are a popular vegetarian-friendly choice. For the healthiest options, ask for whole-wheat pasta or whole-wheat crusts on pizza. Pizza can even be a dairy-free option if you ask them to hold the cheese and add extra tomato sauce and lots of vegetables.

1. Eat something raw before you go out to fill you up.
2. Drink two quarts of water before you go out.
3. Almost all restaurants will offer a side salad. Ask for lemon wedges and some olive oil.
4. Make up a laminated 3X5 card to give to the waiter at restaurants. Specify on the card that you eat only plant-based foods such as fruits, vegetables, leafy greens, nuts, seeds, and sprouts. This eliminates all the guesswork and lengthy explanations in communicating with the wait staff. The best part? I've had some fabulous meals! And, more often than not, the chef has come out of the kitchen and visited my table to make sure the meal was to my satisfaction.
5. Ask the waiter to ask the chef if he/she can make up a special raw/vegan entrée for you. Some chefs have been trained in raw/vegan and never get to practice it due to lack of demand. They may enjoy the challenge to be creative and have a change of pace. You might be pleasantly surprised!

Growing Your Own Living Foods

Success Going to Parties!

Quite often people are hesitant to invite a vegetarian over for dinner, since it can feel very intimidating. Put their minds at ease by saying you can fill up on the side dishes and a salad, which is available at almost every table. You can also offer to bring an entrée or side dish.
If your host does not know you are a vegetarian, it's best to tell them when you first receive the invitation. This allows them to make sure there are food options for you, and in the case of a formal dinner, it prevents them from being offended when they notice you avoiding their lovingly prepared meat entrée.

So, do I hesitate when I am presented with the opportunity to eat out or at a friend's house? Absolutely not! Healthy choices can be found almost anywhere, life is for living to the fullest, and people are for loving to the utmost.

1. Eat something raw before you go to the party.
2. Drink two quarts of water before you go to the party.
3. Prepare a raw dish ahead of time and take it with you to share with others.
4. Eat only what you brought plus any raw salads and veggie sticks at the party.
5. Get involved in the local raw food community and go to raw meetups!
6. Hold raw potlucks in your home!

Success at Work!

1. Prepare two quarts of green smoothie before you leave the house. Use ice to keep it cool. Put them in mason jars and take it with you to work in a cooler.
2. Put some carrot sticks and celery sticks in the cooler for snacks.
3. Google raw restaurants near your place of work.
4. Consider bringing a second blender in to work and leaving it there. Bring fruits and veggies in to work each day and make smoothies in the office.

Growing Your Own Living Foods

Success When You Travel!

I recently went to a conference where all the attendees ate their meals at the host hotel. As soon as I arrived, I explained my eating habits to the server. Every meal after that, the kitchen made a special dish just for me. While others were served what we jokingly called "rubber chicken" dishes, I was served a colorful dish with a host of vegetables, wild rice, or pastas. When compared, the other attendees said they would have preferred mine. At any choice hotel or special event, tell the server as soon as possible what your food requirements are. They usually will be very accommodating.

Here are a number of other road-tested travel tips for vegetarians:
* Carry food with you, such as your favorite granóla or superfood bars, fruit, and chopped vegetables. Before traveling, stop at a supermarket or health food store to stock up on fruit, nuts, and distilled or purified water, so you'll always have a healthy snack on hand.
* Fast-food restaurants should be avoided when possible, but even on a road trip with fast food at every turn, you can still make the right choices. At Subway my favorite is the 6" veggie delight with whole- wheat bread, vegetables, and a spritz of olive oil and vinegar. Vegetarian fare is also available at Taco Bell, Burger King, Chipotle, and select McDonald's and Quizno's, just to name a few.
* When you travel, search your navigation system or the Internet for local Whole Foods or Wild Oats stores. Both stores have deli counters and extensive salad bars where you can find everything from Indian curries to vegan potato salad.
* When choosing accommodations, request a room with a kitchenette or at least a refrigerator. This allows you to shop for food in grocery stores, save money, and know what you are eating.
* Do your homework before traveling to another country. Be prepared to speak your food requests in the native tongue. You don't even need a bilingual dictionary, just enter a few basic, key phrases into Google to translate, such as "I am a vegetarian." "I do not eat meat or fish. Which of these dishes can I eat?" "Is there a vegetarian restaurant near here?" If you have a hard time speaking another language, translate your requests onto a note card and carry it with you.

Growing Your Own Living Foods

* When in a different country, understand that what you are putting into your mouth may not be what you think. A good rule of thumb is to never eat from a street vendor! Instead, pull out the supply of snacks you packed from home.
* Web sites such as www.HappyCow.com list healthy restaurants, health food stores, and even vegetarian/vegan bed and breakfasts around the world.

1. Sprout bags work great for growing sprouts while on the road. They fold up flat so they do not take up any space and there is no glass to break. You can grow sprouts in your hotel room by hanging your sprout bag up by the shower curtain.
2. EasySprouter comes with a flat lid with holes in it designed specifically for growing sprouts while travelling. This way your sprouts can still breath with no danger of spilling.
3. Plan ahead. Bring carrot and celery sticks with you when you travel.
4. Google raw restaurants, juice bars, health food stores, or Whole Foods at your destination.
5. Bring superfood blue-green algae WildBars and BGBars.
6. Drink lots of water when flying. Air travel causes dehydration.
7. When traveling abroad take probiotics every day for two weeks prior to your trip. This prevents Montezuma's revenge.

Tips!

1. Resist the temptation to critique the Standard American Diet (SAD) people around you. Instead, be loving, hugging, joking, energize, peaceful, non-violent communicators,
2. Be accepting. Be an example. Concentrate on your own self. You have unlimited power over one person.
3. You will have more time and energy so, you need to find a new hobby (write a book, art lessons, learn a new language, spend more time with your children, garden, yoga, meditate, take interesting educational courses, voice lessons.)

Growing Your Own Living Foods

Chapter 11 – How Much Should I Grow?

Sprout Schedule

How many sprouts you should grow depends upon what else you are including in your diet such as bread, dairy, cheese, milk, eggs, fish, coffee, soda, beer, wine, etc. If your question is "how much wheatgrass and sprouts do I need to grow for a family of 2 *if we are 100% hard core, 100% raw vegan and 100% on the Hippocrates program including green drinks and wheatgrass implants* " then here is the formula:

Sprout (approx.)	Plant per week	Crop Starts
Adzuki	1 cup	½ cup every other day
Mung	1 cup	½ cup every other day
Green lentils	1 cup	½ cup every other day
Red lentils	1 cup	½ cup every other day
Fenugreek	1 cup	½ cup every other day
Alfalfa	¼ cup	2 Tbs. every third day
Broccoli	¼ cup	2 Tbs. every third day
Cabbage	¼ cup	2 Tbs. every third day
Clover	¼ cup	2 Tbs. every third day
Garlic	2 Tbs	1 Tbs. every third day
Onion	2 Tbs	1 Tbs. every third day
Radish	¼ cup	2 Tbs. every third day
Wheatgrass	8 – 10"X 10" trays	1 tray a day
Sunflower	8 – 10"X 10" trays	1 tray a day
Pea Shoots	10 – 10"X 10" trays	1 tray a day
Buckwheat	1 – 10"X 10" tray	1 tray a week

Some types of sprouts are grown just for eating such as adzuki, mung beans, lentils, fenugreek, garbanzo, alfalfa, clover, broccoli, radish, onion, beet, garlic, cabbage, and buckwheat. Other types of sprouts we both juice and we eat like sunflower and pea. Wheatgrass is grown only for juicing since we do not have the digestive enzymes sufficient to liquefy the tough grass blades.

Growing Your Own Living Foods

Ideally, at least half of your diet should be sprouts. If you eat this way the average person will need about four cups of sprouts per day. That is, two cups for lunch and two cups for dinner. But, not all your sprouts should be of a single type. You want to have a variety of sprouts in your diet. Every plant mines different minerals as it grows. By having a variety of sprouts in your diet you will be getting a more balanced nutritional profile. One tablespoon each of perhaps eight to ten different sprouts will add up to about two cups.

It only takes one square foot of your kitchen countertop space to grow five pounds of food in the form of sprouts growing in Mason jars. You could have nine to twelve Mason jars all lined up on a bamboo dish drying rack with each one growing a different type of sprout. Every sprout mines different minerals as it grows. By having a variety of sprouts daily you will insure you are getting a complete and balanced nutritional diet.

Yields

You may not get the kind of yields described below on your first attempt. But, you will get better at it over time with practice.

Wheatgrass

We only juice wheatgrass. A 10" X 10" tray will yield up to one pound of wheatgrass. This will produce up to nine ounces of wheatgrass juice when using a good quality auger style juicer. What you are not going to use right away you can store them dry in the refrigerator in a covered container where they will keep for up to five days. But, fresh is best so I recommend growing in smaller trays so you have less wheatgrass stored in the refrigerator for a shorter period of time.

Sunflower Sprouts

We both juice and we eat sunflower sprouts. A 10" X 10" tray will yield up to 28 ounces of sunflower sprouts. This will produce up to 21 ounces of sunflower sprout juice when using a good quality auger style juicer. What you are not going to use right away you can store them dry in the refrigerator in a covered container where they will keep for up to five days. But, fresh is best so I recommend growing in smaller trays so you have less sunflower sprouts stored in the refrigerator for a shorter period of time.

Pea Shoot Sprouts

We both juice and we eat pea shoot sprouts. A 10" X 10" tray will yield up to 20 ounces of pea shoot sprouts. This will produce up to 15 ounces of pea shoot sprout juice when using a good quality auger style juicer. What you are not going to use right away you can store them dry in the refrigerator in a covered container where they will keep for up to five days. But, fresh is best so I recommend growing in smaller trays so you have less sunflower sprouts stored in the refrigerator for a shorter period of time.

Buckwheat Sprouts

We only eat buckwheat sprouts. A 10" X 10" tray will yield up to 28 ounces of buckwheat sprouts. What you are not going to use right away you can store them dry in the refrigerator in a covered container where they will keep for up to two days. But, fresh is best so I recommend growing in smaller trays so you have less sunflower sprouts stored in the refrigerator for a shorter period of time.

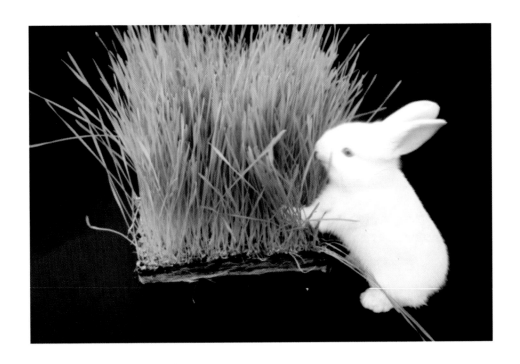

Chapter 12 – Troubleshooting

Mold

Mold in your wheatgrass or sprouts can be caused by any one of the following:

1. Not enough air flow. You need a little gentle air flow. A ceiling fan nearby set on low speed is ideal. If you see the blades of grass moving as a result of the action of the fan, it is either on too high a speed setting or it is positioned too close to the grass. Just move the fan a little further away or slow down the fan speed. This one thing will resolve 90% of mold problems.
2. Temperature is greater than 75 degrees F. This means the best place to grow is indoors in air conditioning.
3. Humidity is greater than 50%. This means growing indoors in air conditioning.
4. Trays are not drained well. Use only trays with holes on a rack or otherwise supported so they are not sitting in their own drain water. Do not water from the bottom up. Use only organic potting mix.
5. Trays and sprouting containers are not clean. Clean every nook and cranny with a good natural organic dish detergent or grapefruit seed extract and water solution after each use.
6. Seeds are old and/or bad. Try changing your seeds out for new and/or from a different source.

If you do get a little mold on your wheatgrass you can usually rinse it off with cool water. However, if the blades of grass have turned brown that part should be cut off and discarded.

Wheatgrass Nausea

Nausea from drinking wheatgrass juice can be caused by several things:

1. Mold. Make sure you rinse your wheatgrass before juicing to wash away any mold. Then, it is ok to use.

2. Old wheatgrass. The older the wheatgrass the more bitter it gets. Harvest your wheatgrass while it is still young just at the beginning of the jointing stage. Every day after the jointing stage it ages 40 years. Juice as soon as possible after cutting.
3. No direct sunlight during growing. Allow plenty of indirect sunlight and artificial, full spectrum lighting. When exposed to direct sun your wheatgrass will get too bitter.
4. Drinking too much in one sitting. Limit your wheatgrass shots to 2 ounces (or less) at a time.
5. Wheatgrass juice is a powerful detoxifier. It is not meant to be a flavorful recreational drink. It is medicine. Wheatgrass juice cleans you out top to bottom like Roto-Rooter™. It sucks toxins, poisons, pollution, and heavy metals right out of your tissues. The more nauseous it makes you, the more you need it.
6. Because of the strong detoxifying effect it is best to drink wheatgrass juice on an empty stomach.
7. If you cannot drink it you can still do wheatgrass implants instead.

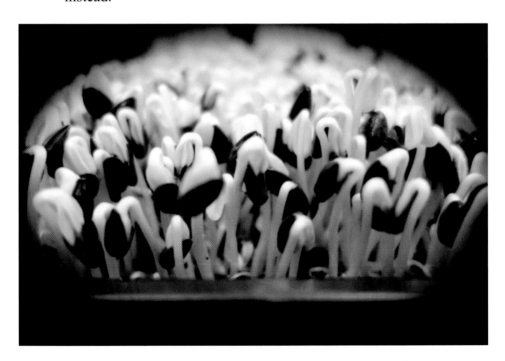

Growing Your Own Living Foods

Yellow Wheatgrass Blades

This usually means not enough light

Uneven Wheatgrass Blade Growth

Uneven wheatgrass blades usually means or not enough water or not enough water. Water twice a day heavy just until the tray starts to drip. Use trays with holes in the bottom and support your trays so they do not sit in their own drain water.

Bugs in Your Wheatgrass

Here is what you can do for bugs:

1.   Take all fruit off the counter and keep it in the refrigerator. Bugs come for the fruit first and then they set up home in the wheatgrass.
2.   Keep a fan on low nearby. Their tiny little wings cannot handle the turbulence.
3.   Using a vacuum cleaner, wave the upoulstry wand over the wheatgrass trays to suck up all the bugs.
4.   Hang up fly paper near the wheatgrass trays.

Seeds Do Not Germinate

This could be caused by several things:

1. Bad seeds
2. Soaking too long

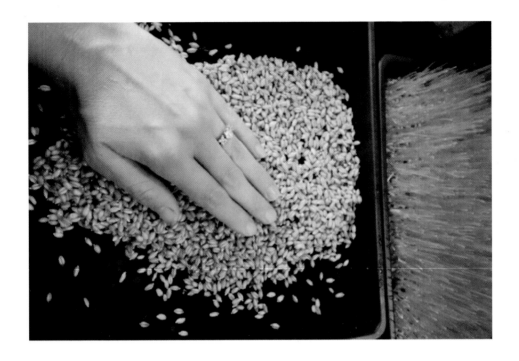

Growing Your Own Living Foods

<u>Chapter 13 – Sprout Studies</u>

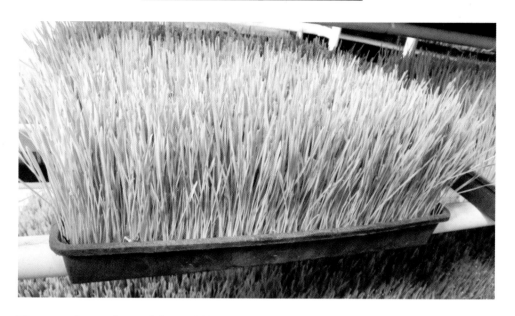

Here are just a few of the published clinical research studies on the amazing power of fresh wheatgrass juice and sprouts:

(1) Effect of wheat grass juice in supportive care of terminally ill cancer patients—A tertiary cancer centre experience from India.

Dey S., Sarkar R., Ghosh P, et al. 2006 J. Clin. Onc. 24:18;2006:8634

Background: Researchers have previously shown that when animals with abnormally low levels of red blood cells and low hemoglobin (anemia) are given a solution containing chlorophyll and related compounds, the animals more rapidly recover from their anemia. Anemia is a common occurrence in patients undergoing chemotherapy to treat cancer, though it may also occur simply as a consequence of long-standing cancer. Anemia in this context is a source of significant suffering for patients and may require blood transfusions in severe cases.

Clinical Trial: Initially stimulated by this great variety of health benefits of wheatgrass juice, a team of researchers from the Palliative Care Unit of the Netaji Subhash Chandra Bose Cancer Research Institute in India studied the effectiveness of wheatgrass in 400 terminally ill solid-organ cancer patients (age range, 22 - 87 years) examined over a period of 3 years. The study focused on changes in the haemoglobin level, serum protein and performance status, in particular noting the capacity of wheatgrass juice to improve quality of life.

Fresh juice was prepared from the leaves and roots of 5-day-old wheatgrass, and 30 ml doses were administered daily for 6 months. The sites of the treated cancers were: lung (25% of patients), breast (20%), oesophagus (11%), colon (9%), ovary (8%), liver (6%), stomach (6%), and other (15%).

Conclusion: The results in 348 patients, after exclusion of 50 patients requiring transfusion support, were significant improvements in haemoglobin, total protein and albumin levels, and a performance status enhanced from 50% to 70% on the Karnovsky Scale (this runs from 100 to 0, where 100 is "perfect" health and 0 is death.) The authors concluded that wheatgrass juice is an excellent alternative to blood transfusion.

(2) Wheat grass juice may improve hematological toxicity related to chemotherapy in breast cancer patients: a pilot study.

Bar-Sela G, Tsalic M, Fried G, Goldberg H. Nutr Cancer. 2007;58(1):43-48.

Background: Chemotherapy has greatly improved our ability to treat cancer, but the treatment comes with a physical cost. One of the most troubling and dangerous side effects of chemotherapy is hematological toxicity. Chemotherapy is designed to kill human cells. Ideally it would kill just cancer cells, but the chemotherapeutic drugs are not always that selective and may destroy healthy, important cells. One of the most commonly affected cells are those of the blood. When chemotherapy destroys red and white blood cells and platelets, it causes anemia, immune system deficits, and blood clotting disorders, respectively.

Clinical Study: Cancer researchers in Israel studied the effect that wheatgrass juice has on patients undergoing chemotherapy for breast cancer. They followed 60 patients receiving cytotoxic (cell-killing) chemotherapy; approximately half the patients received wheatgrass juice and the other half simply received routine care. Significantly fewer patients in the wheatgrass juice group had serious events of blood toxicity than the standard care group. The wheatgrass juice group had fewer instances of neutropenic fever, leucopenia with infection, and prolonged neutropenia (low white blood cells). Hemoglobin levels were negatively affected by chemotherapy in both groups, but to a much lower degree in the wheatgrass juice group. Patients taking wheatgrass needed fewer drugs to support blood cell number and function. The one reported side effect of wheatgrass juice was that a majority of patients had difficulty consuming the juice because of its strong odor and taste. This led to increased nausea.

Conclusion: Wheatgrass juice, when taken along with chemotherapy, helped maintain healthier levels of blood cells and reduced the need for additional supportive medications. The use of wheatgrass juice may be limited because of the strong flavor of the substance in its raw state.

(3) The role of iron chelation activity of wheat grass juice in blood transfusion requirement of intermediate thalassaemia.

Mukhopadhyay. S., Mukhopadhyay. A., Gupta. P., Kar. M., Ghosh. A. 2007 Am. Soc. Hematol. Ann.

Background: The authors noted there was no satisfactory explanation for reduced blood transfusion requirements in thalassemia major patients treated with fresh wheatgrass juice. (Marwaha et al) Thalassemias are diseases of abnormal hemoglobin, the oxygen carrying protein of the blood. There is a range of severities in the disease from relatively mild to fatal. In some instances frequent blood transfusions are necessary to provide patients with enough functional hemoglobin. Unfortunately since transfused blood carries iron, the patient accumulates excessive levels of iron in the body. Too much iron is toxic to the body, particularly the liver and nervous system.

Clinical Trial: 30mls of fresh wheatgrass juice extracted from 6 week old wheatgrass plants was given daily to 200 thalassemia intermedia patients over 6 months. They included E-beta thalassemia (160 patients), E-thalassemia, (30 patients) and 10 patients with Sickle thalassemia. Significant iron chelating activity comparable with a standard pharmaceutical chelator, desferrioxamine, was observed. Mean hemoglobin levels rose from 6.2gm% to 7.8gm% (26% increase). Serum ferritin levels decreased significantly and the 24 patients requiring incremental blood transfusion enjoyed an increased interval between transfusions. The authors concluded that wheatgrass juice is an effective alternative to blood transfusion in thalassemia intermedia patients and its use should be encouraged.

Conclusion: The use of orally consumed wheatgrass juice improved hemoglobin values in patients with intermediate thalassemia. It also possibly reduced the need for blood transfusions. Wheatgrass juice dose-dependently chelates iron, which could be helpful in patients who require frequent transfusions.

(4) The role of iron chelation activity of wheat grass juice in patients with myelodysplastic syndrome.

Mukhopadhyay. S., Basak. J., Kar. M., Mandal. S., Mukhopadhyay. A. 2009. J. Clin. Oncology 2009:7012

Background: Myelodysplastic syndrome describes any number of conditions in which the bone marrow does not produce enough blood cells. In cases where red blood cell number drops too low, patients require blood transfusion to add additional red blood cells. The blood that is transfused carries iron and, when numerous transfusions are given, the patient may have harmful and excessive levels of iron in the body. Medications that bind to and remove metals, such as iron, are called chelators. Sometimes chelators are prescribed to counter the toxic effects of too much iron. Lastly, ferritin is a protein that stores iron—the level of ferritin correlates with the level of iron in the body.
Clinical Trial: Physicians collected a cohort of 20 patients with severe myelodysplastic syndrome who required repeated blood transfusions. They administered 30 mL of fresh wheatgrass juice made from 5-7 day old leaves daily for 6 months. The wheatgrass juice had two intriguing

properties. The first was that it had the ability to chelate or bind to iron. Also, mean serum ferritin levels, (an indicator of the amount of iron in the blood), fell from 2,250 to 950 and the mean interval between transfusion increased. This effect was comparable to a medically prescribed iron chelator, desferrioxamine, suggesting that the juice was able to clear iron from the body.

Conclusion: Wheatgrass juice dose-dependently chelates iron on a par with prescription chelators. The juice also apparently reduced the iron burden of patients who receive repeated blood transfusions. The authors concluded that "wheatgrass juice is an effective iron chelator, and its use in reducing serum ferritin should be encouraged in myelodysplastic syndrome and other diseases where repeated blood transfusion is required."

(5) Evidence for an unidentified growth factor(s) from alfalfa and other plant sources. Lakhanpal,R., Davis, J., Typpo, J., Briggs, G. 1966. J, Nutr. 89(3):341-346

Factor(s) important for growth in guinea pigs were found in alfalfa, broccoli and grass clippings. They may or may not be related to the 'grass juice factor', but are organic in nature since they are not found in ash.

(6) Wheat grass juice reduces transfusion requirements in patients with thalassemia major: a pilot study. Marwaha, R., Bansal, D., Kaur, S., Trehan A.2004. Indian Ped. 41:716-720

Patients with thalassemia consuming wheat grass juice on a daily basis reduced on average their requirements for blood transfusion. Families raised and prepared the wheat grass at home and a comparison was made with the requirements of the patient in the preceding year. In nearly all patients the mean interval between visits increased and the blood transfused decreased during the wheat grass period. The mechanism involved is unknown.

Growing Your Own Living Foods

(7) Growth stimulating properties of grass juice. Kohler G, Elvehjem C, Hart E. Science. 1936. 445

Growth of rats increases on a diet of milk produced on summer pasture compared with milk produced from winter feeding conditions. i.e. fodder. When grass juice was added to the winter milk diet, growth doubled from 2 to 4 grams a day. It was evident there are important water-soluble substances in the juice that directly stimulate growth when added to winter milk.

(8) Wheat grass juice in the treatment of active distal ulcerative colitis: a randomized double-blind placebo-controlled trial.

Scand J Gastroenterol. 2002 Apr;37(4):444-9.
Ben-Arye E, Goldin E, Wengrower D, Stamper A, Kohn R, Berry E.
Source
Dept. of Family Medicine, The Bruce Rappaport Faculty of Medicine, The Technion, Israel Institute of Technology, Haifa. eranben@netvision.net.il
Abstract
BACKGROUND:
The use of wheat grass (Triticum aestivum) juice for treatment of various gastrointestinal and other conditions had been suggested by its proponents for more than 30 years, but was never clinically assessed in a controlled trial. A preliminary unpublished pilot study suggested efficacy of wheat grass juice in the treatment of ulcerative colitis (UC).
METHODS:
A randomized, double-blind, placebo-controlled study. One gastroenterology unit in a tertiary hospital and three study coordinating centers in three major cities in Israel. Twenty-three patients diagnosed clinically and sigmoidoscopically with active distal UC were randomly allocated to receive either 100 cc of wheat grass juice, or a matching placebo, daily for 1 month. Efficacy of treatment was assessed by a 4-fold disease activity index that included rectal bleeding and number of bowel movements as determined from patient diary records, a sigmoidoscopic evaluation, and global assessment by a physician.
RESULTS:
Twenty-one patients completed the study, and full information was

available on 19 of them. Treatment with wheat grass juice was associated with significant reductions in the overall disease activity index (P=0.031) and in the severity of rectal bleeding (P = 0.025). No serious side effects were found. Fresh extract of wheat grass demonstrated a prominent tracing in cyclic voltammetry methodology, presumably corresponding to four groups of compounds that exhibit anti-oxidative properties.
CONCLUSION:
Wheat grass juice appeared effective and safe as a single or adjuvant treatment of active distal UC.

(9) Wheat Sprout Extract Induces Changes On 20S Proteasomes Functionality

Amici M, Bonfili L, Spina M, Cecarini V, Calzuola I, Marsili V, Angeletti M, Fioretti E, Tacconi R, Gianfranceschi GL, Eleuteri AM.
University of Camerino, Department of Biology M.C.A., 62032 Camerino (MC), Italy.

Wheat sprouts contain a very high level of organic phosphates and a powerful cocktail of different molecules such as enzymes, reducing glycosides and polyphenols. The antioxidant properties of wheat sprouts have been widely documented and it has been shown that they **are able to protect DNA against free-radicals mediated oxidative damage**. Furthermore, we have recently reported on the effects of several polyphenols on 20S proteasomes, underlying the dual role of epigallocatechin-3-gallate as **an antioxidant and a proteasome effector in cancer cells**. The aim of this study was to investigate the effects of wheat sprout extracts on 20S proteasome functionality. Wheat sprout extracts have been analysed and characterized for their polyphenolic content using the Folin-Ciocalteau reagent and RP-HPLC technique. Comparing our data with a polyphenol standard mixture we identified five different polyphenols: gallic acid, epigallocatechin-3-gallate, epigallocatechin, epicatechin and catechin. The treatment of isolated 20S proteasomes with the extract induced a gradual inhibition of all the tested components, ChT-L, T-L, PGPH and BrAAP, in both the complexes. At low extract concentration a slight activation of the enzyme was evident only for the BrAAP component of the constitutive enzyme and the ChT-L activity of the immunoproteasome. Beta-casein degradation rate decreased, particularly with the immunoproteasome. **Human Colon adenocarcinoma (Caco) cells, stimulated with 12-O-tetradecanoylphorbol-13-acetate, showed activation of the 20S proteasome activities at short incubation times and an increase in intracellular oxidative proteins.** Cells treatment with wheat sprout extract led to proteasome inhibition in unstimulated cells and attenuated the effects mediated by TPA. Finally, exposure to the extract affected the expression levels of pro-apoptotic proteins.

(10) Wheat Grass Juice May Improve Hematological Toxicity Related to Chemotherapy in Breast Cancer Patients: A Pilot Study

DOI:10.1080/01635580701308083
Gil Bar-Selaa, Medy Tsalica, Getta Frieda & Hadassah Goldberga
pages 43-48
Published online: 05 Dec 2007

Myelotoxicity induced by chemotherapy may become life-threatening. Neutropenia may be prevented by granulocyte colony-stimulating factors (GCSF), and epoetin may prevent anemia, but both cause substantial side effects and increased costs. According to non-established data, wheat grass juice (WGJ) may prevent myelotoxicity when applied with chemotherapy. In this prospective matched control study, 60 patients with breast carcinoma on chemotherapy were enrolled and assigned to an intervention or control arm. Those in the intervention arm (A) were given 60 cc of WGJ orally daily during the first three cycles of chemotherapy, while those in the control arm (B) received only regular supportive therapy. Premature termination of treatment, dose reduction, and starting GCSF or epoetin were considered as "censoring events." Response rate to chemotherapy was calculated in patients with evaluable disease. Analysis of the results showed that five censoring events occurred in Arm A and 15 in Arm B (P = 0.01). Of the 15 events in Arm B, 11 were related to hematological events. No reduction in response rate was observed in patients who could be assessed for response. Side effects related to WGJ were minimal, including worsening of nausea in six patients, causing cessation of WGJ intake. In conclusion, it was found that WGJ taken during FAC chemotherapy may reduce myelotoxicity, dose reductions, and need for GCSF support, without diminishing efficacy of chemotherapy. These preliminary results need confirmation in a phase III study.

(11) Wheat Grass Juice in the Treatment of Active Distal Ulcerative Colitis: A Randomized Double-blind Placebo-controlled Trial

2002, Vol. 37, No. 4 , Pages 444-449 (doi:10.1080/003655202317316088)
E. Ben-Arye, E. Goldin, D. Wengrower, A. Stamper, R. Kohn and E. Berry

Background: The use of wheat grass (Triticum aestivum) juice for treatment of various gastrointestinal and other conditions had been suggested by its proponents for more than 30 years, but was never clinically assessed in a controlled trial. A preliminary unpublished pilot study suggested efficacy of wheat grass juice in the treatment of ulcerative colitis (UC). Methods: A randomized, double-blind, placebo controlled study. One gastroenterology unit in a tertiary hospital and three study coordinating centers in three major cities in Israel. Twenty-three patients diagnosed clinically and sigmoidoscopically with active distal UC were randomly allocated to receive either 100 cc of wheat grass juice, or a matching placebo, daily for 1 month. Efficacy of treatment was assessed by a 4-fold disease activity index that included rectal bleeding and number of bowel movements as determined from patient diary records, a sigmoidoscopic evaluation, and global assessment by a physician. Results. Twenty-one patients completed the study, and full information was available on 19 of them. Treatment with wheat grass juice was associated with significant reductions in the overall disease activity index (P = 0.031) and in the severity of rectal bleeding (P = 0.025). No serious side effects were found. Fresh extract of wheat grass demonstrated a prominent tracing in cyclic voltammetry methodology, presumably corresponding to four groups of compounds that exhibit anti-oxidative properties. Conclusion. Wheat grass juice appeared effective and safe as a single or adjuvant treatment of active distal UC.

Growing Your Own Living Foods

Sulforaphane (derived from broccoli sprouts) treatment of autism spectrum disorder (ASD)

Pnas.org - October 28, 2014, vol. 111 no. 43 > Kanwaljit Singh, 15550–15555, doi: 10.1073/pnas.1416940111

Kanwaljit Singh[a,b], Susan L. Connors[a], Eric A. Macklin[c], Kirby D. Smith[d], Jed W. Fahey[e], Paul Talalay[e,1], and Andrew W. Zimmerman[a,b,1]

Autism spectrum disorder (ASD), encompassing impaired communication and social interaction, and repetitive stereotypic behavior and language, affects 1–2% of predominantly male individuals and is an enormous medical and economic problem for which there is no documented, mechanism-based treatment. In a placebo-controlled, randomized, double-blind clinical trial, daily oral administration for 18 wk of the phytochemical sulforaphane (derived from broccoli sprouts) to 29 young men with ASD substantially (and reversibly) improved behavior compared with 15 placebo recipients. Behavior was quantified by both parents/caregivers and physicians by three widely accepted measures. Sulforaphane, which showed negligible toxicity, was selected because it upregulates genes that protect aerobic cells against oxidative stress, inflammation, and DNA-damage, all of which are prominent and possibly mechanistic characteristics of ASD.

Autism spectrum disorder (ASD), characterized by both impaired communication and social interaction, and by stereotypic behavior, affects about 1 in 68, predominantly males. The medico-economic burdens of ASD are enormous, and no recognized treatment targets the core features of ASD. In a placebo-controlled, double-blind, randomized trial, young men (aged 13–27) with moderate to severe ASD received the phytochemical sulforaphane (n = 29)—derived from broccoli sprout extracts—or indistinguishable placebo (n = 15). The effects on behavior of daily oral doses of sulforaphane (50–150 μmol) for 18 wk, followed by 4 wk without treatment, were quantified by three widely accepted behavioral measures completed by parents/caregivers and physicians: the Aberrant Behavior Checklist (ABC), Social Responsiveness Scale (SRS), and Clinical Global Impression Improvement Scale (CGI-I). Initial scores for

Growing Your Own Living Foods

ABC and SRS were closely matched for participants assigned to placebo and sulforaphane. After 18 wk, participants receiving placebo experienced minimal change (<3.3%), whereas those receiving sulforaphane showed substantial declines (improvement of behavior): 34% for ABC (P < 0.001, comparing treatments) and 17% for SRS scores (P = 0.017). On CGI-I, a significantly greater number of participants receiving sulforaphane had improvement in social interaction, abnormal behavior, and verbal communication (P = 0.015–0.007). Upon discontinuation of sulforaphane, total scores on all scales rose toward pretreatment levels. Dietary sulforaphane, of recognized low toxicity, was selected for its capacity to reverse abnormalities that have been associated with ASD, including oxidative stress and lower antioxidant capacity, depressed glutathione synthesis, reduced mitochondrial function and oxidative phosphorylation, increased lipid peroxidation, and neuroinflammmation.

Cancer Protection Compound Abundant in Broccoli Sprouts

hopkinsmedicine.org - September 15, 1997

JOHNS HOPKINS SCIENTISTS have found a new and highly concentrated source of sulforaphane, a compound they identified in 1992 that helps mobilize the body's natural cancer-fighting resources and reduces risk of developing cancer.

"Three-day-old broccoli sprouts consistently contain 20 to 50 times the amount of chemoprotective compounds found in mature broccoli heads, and may offer a simple, dietary means of chemically reducing cancer risk," says Paul Talalay, M.D., J.J. Abel Distinguished Service Professor of Pharmacology.

Talalay's research team fed extracts of the sprouts to groups of 20 female rats for five days, and exposed them and a control group that had not received the extracts to a carcinogen, dimethylbenzanthracene. The rats that received the extracts developed fewer tumors, and those that did get tumors had smaller growths that took longer to develop.

In a paper published in tomorrow's issue of the Proceedings of the

Growing Your Own Living Foods

National Academy of Sciences, Talalay and his coworkers describe their successful efforts to build on their 1992 discovery of sulforaphane's chemoprotective properties. Work described in the study is the subject of issued and pending patents.

A systematic search for dietary sources of compounds that increase resistance to cancer-causing agents led the Hopkins group to focus on naturally occurring compounds in edible plants that mobilize Phase 2 detoxification enzymes. These enzymes neutralize highly reactive, dangerous forms of cancer-causing chemicals before they can damage DNA and promote cancer.

Sulforaphane "is a very potent promoter of Phase 2 enzymes," says Jed Fahey, plant physiologist and manager of the Brassica Chemoprotection Laboratory at Hopkins, and broccoli contains unusually high levels of glucoraphanin, the naturally-occurring precursor of sulforaphane.

However, tests reported in the new study showed that glucoraphanin levels were highly variable in broccoli samples, and there was no way to tell which broccoli plants had the most without sophisticated chemical analysis.

"Even if that were possible, people would still have to eat unreasonably large quantities of broccoli to get any significant promotion of Phase 2 enzymes," Talalay says.

Clinical studies are currently under way to see if eating a few tablespoons of the sprouts daily can supply the same degree of chemoprotection as one to two pounds of broccoli eaten weekly. The sprouts look and taste something like alfalfa sprouts, according to Talalay.

Talalay founded the Brassica Chemoprotection Laboratory, a Hopkins center that focuses on identifying chemoprotective nutrients and finding ways to maximize their effects. Brassica is a plant genus more commonly known as the mustard family, and includes in addition to broccoli, Brussels sprouts, cabbage, kale, cauliflower and turnips.

Growing Your Own Living Foods

"Man-made compounds that increase the resistance of cells and tissues to carcinogens are currently under development, but will require years of clinical trials to determine safety and efficacy," Talalay notes. "For now, we may get faster and better impact by looking at dietary means of supplying that protection. Eating more fruits and vegetables has long been associated with reduced cancer risk, so it made sense for us to look at vegetables.

"Scientists currently need to continue to develop new ways of detecting and treating cancer once it is established, but it also makes sense to focus more attention on efforts to prevent cancer from arising," he adds.

Fahey and Yuesheng Zhang, M.D., Ph.D., a postdoctoral fellow, are also authors on the PNAS paper.

Work in Talalay's laboratory is supported by the National Cancer Institute, philanthropic contributions to Brassica Chemoprotection Laboratory, and grants from the Cancer Research Foundation of America and the American Institute for Cancer Research.

Talalay is establishing the Brassica Foundation, a foundation that will test and certify chemoprotective vegetables such as sprouts to raise funds for chemoprotection research.

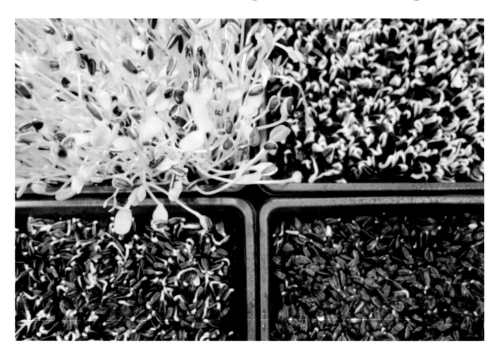